Keto Lunch on a Budget

Cheap and Tasty Keto Recipes to Enjoy Your Lunch and

Save Your Money

Sebastian Booth

Table of contents

Chorizo and Cheese Gofre

Preparation Time **: 10 minutes**

Cooking Time: **20 minutes**

Servings **: 6**

Ingredients

- 6 eggs, separate egg whites and egg yolks
- ½ tsp baking powder
- 6 tbsp almond flour
- 4 tbsp butter, melted
- ¼ tsp salt
- ½ tsp dried rosemary
- 3 tbsp tomato puree
- 3 ounces smoked chorizo, chopped
- **3 ounces cheddar cheese, shredded**

Directions

1. In a mixing bowl, mix egg yolks, almond flour, rosemary, butter, baking powder, and salt. Beat the egg whites until pale and combine with the egg yolk mixture.

2. Grease waffle iron and set over medium heat, add in ¼ cup of the batter and cook for 3 minutes until golden. Repeat with the remaining batter.

3. Place one waffle back to the waffle iron; sprinkle 1 tbsp of tomato puree to the waffle; apply a topping of 1 ounce of cheese and 1 ounce of chorizo. Cover with another waffle Cooking until all the cheese melts.

4. **Do the same with all remaining ingredients.**

Nutrition:

- Calories 244
- Fat 5.7 g
- Carbohydrates 37.1 g
- Sugar 13.2 g
- Protein 11.4 g
- **Cholesterol 10 mg**

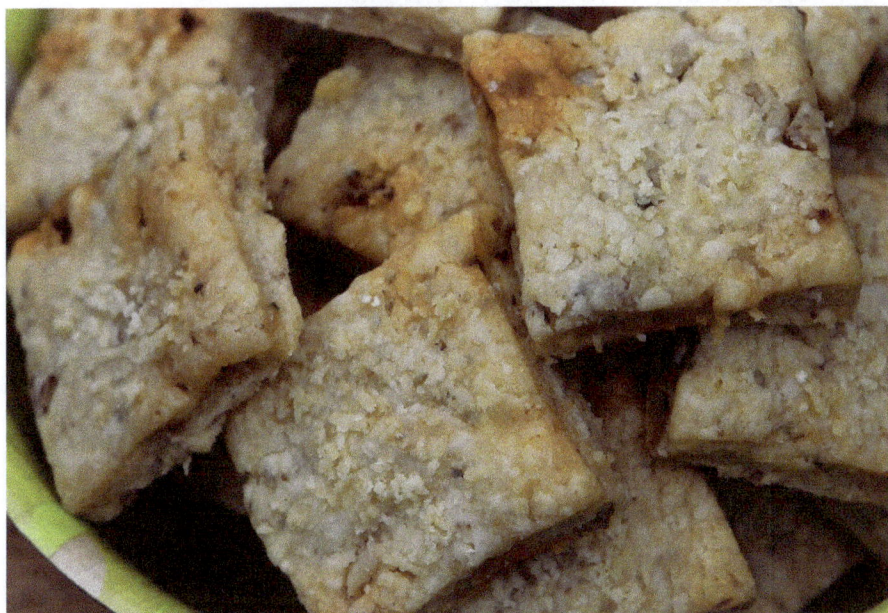

Cheese, Ham and Egg Muffins

Preparation Time **: 10 minutes**

Cooking Time :30 minutes

Servings **: 6**

Ingredients

- 24 slices smoked ham
- 6 eggs, beaten
- Salt and black pepper, to taste
- ¼ cup fresh parsley, chopped
- ¼ cup ricotta cheese
- ¼ cup Brie, chopped

Directions

1. Set oven to 390ºF. Line 2 slices of smoked ham into each greased muffin cup, to circle each mold. In a mixing bowl, mix the rest of the ingredients.
2. Fill ¾ of the ham lined muffin cup with the egg/cheese mixture. Bake for 15 minutes. Serve warm!

Nutrition : Kcal 279 - Carbs 28g - Fat 6g - Protein 17g

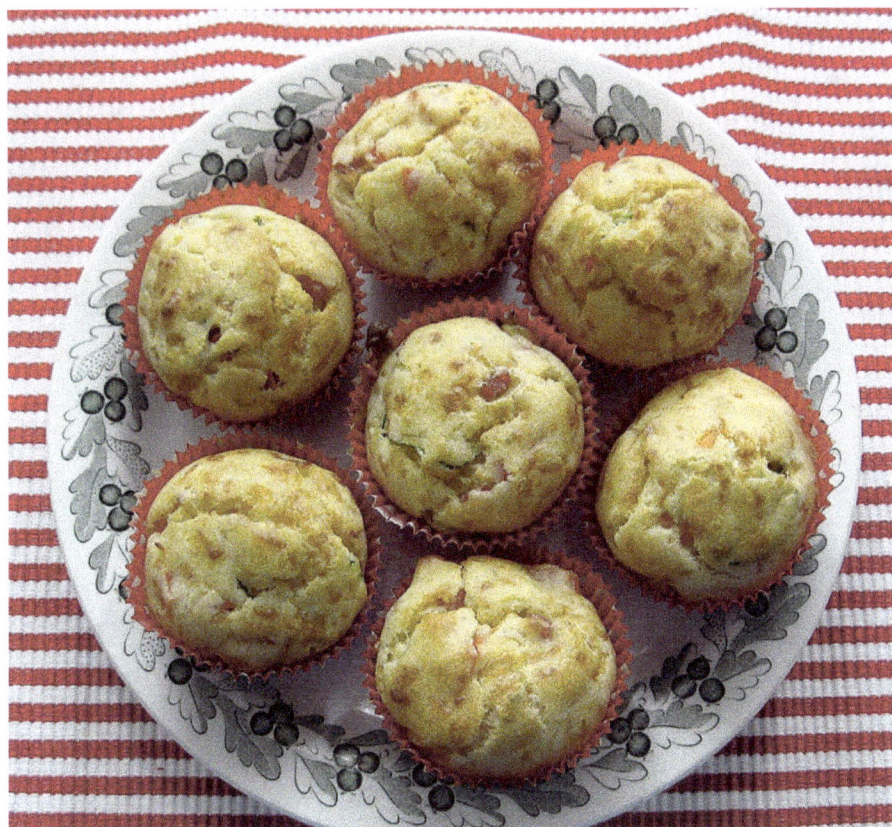

Baked Chicken Legs with Cheesy Spread
Preparation Time: <u>10 minutes</u>

<u>**Cooking Time**</u> :20 minutes

Servings <u>**: 6**</u>

Ingredients

- 4 chicken legs
- ¼ cup goat cheese
- 2 tbsp sour cream
- 1 tbsp butter, softened
- 1 onion, chopped
- **Sea salt and black pepper, to taste**

Directions

1. Preheat oven to 360ºF and season the legs with salt and black pepper.
2. Roast in a greased baking dish for 25-30 minutes until crispy and browned.
3. In a mixing bowl, mix the rest of the ingredients to form the spread. Scatter the spread over the chicken and serve with green salad.

Nutrition:

- Kcal 510
- Carbs 54g
- Fat 21g

- Protein   36g

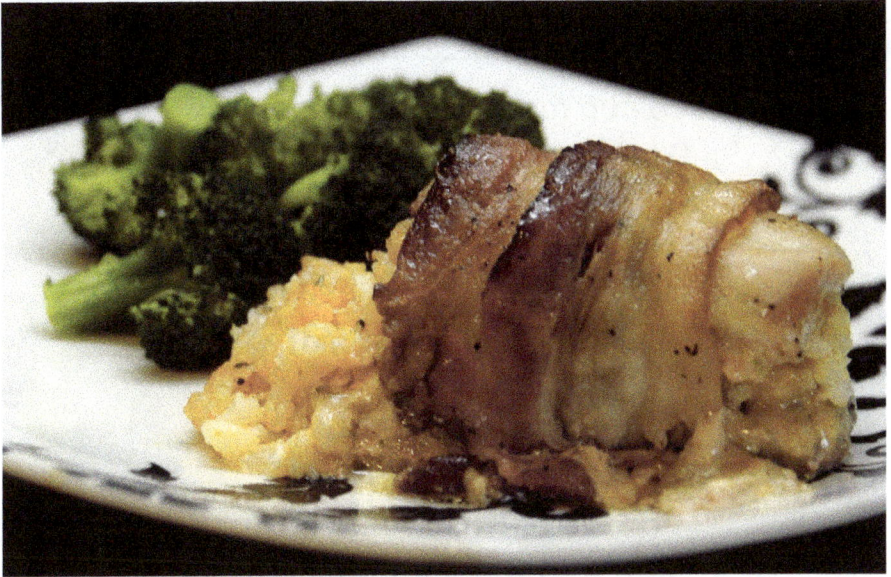

Quattro Formaggio Pizza

Preparation Time: **10 minutes**

Cooking Time :40 minutes

Servings **: 6**

Ingredients

- 1 tbsp olive oil
- ½ cup cheddar cheese, shredded
- 1 ¼ cups mozzarella cheese, shredded
- ½ cup mascarpone cheese
- ½ cup blue cheese
- 2 tbsp sour cream
- 2 garlic cloves, chopped
- 1 red bell pepper, sliced
- 1 green bell pepper, sliced
- 10 cherry tomatoes, halved
- 1 tsp oregano
- **Salt and black pepper, to taste**

Directions

1. In a bowl, mix the cheeses. Set a pan over medium heat and warm olive oil.

2. Spread the cheese mixture on the pan and cook for 5 minutes until cooked through. Scatter garlic and sour cream over the crust.

3. Add in tomatoes and bell peppers Cooking for 2 minutes. Sprinkle with pepper, salt and oregano and serve.

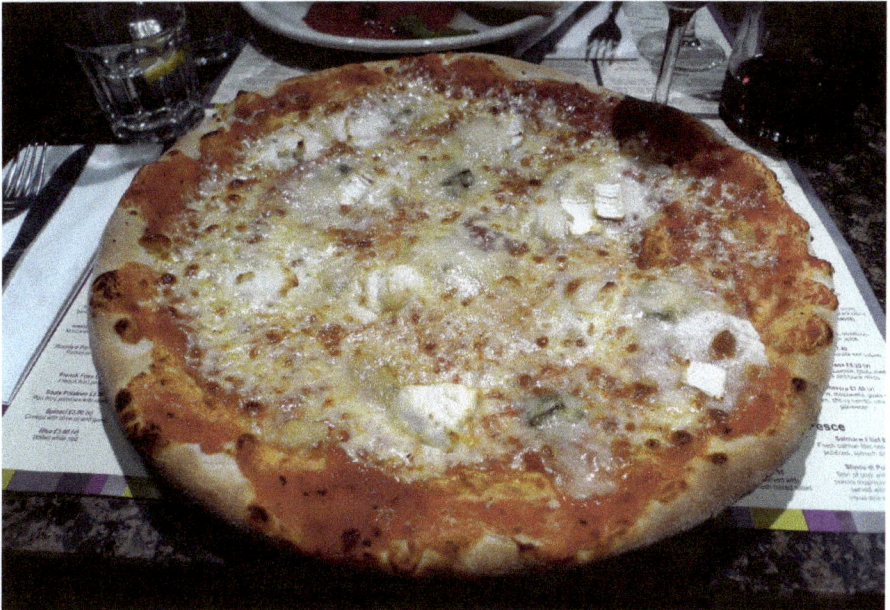

Herbal Green Beans and Chicken

Preparation Time: **15 minutes**

Cooking Time : 35 minutes

Servings: **3**

Ingredients:

- Olive oil (2 tbsp.)
- Trimmed green beans (1 cup)
- Whole chicken breasts (2)
- Cherry tomatoes (8 halve)
- Italian seasoning (1 tbsp.)
- Salt and pepper (1 tsp. of each)

Directions:

1. Warm a skillet using the medium heat setting; add the oil.
2. Sprinkle the chicken with the pepper, Italian seasoning, and salt.
3. Arrange in the skillet for 10 minutes per side – or until thoroughly done.
4. Add the tomatoes and beans. Simmer another 5 to 7 minutes and serve.

Nutrition: Kcal 336 - Carbs 43g - Fat 13g - Protein 15g

Bacon Balls with Brie Cheese

Preparation Time: **10 minutes**

Cooking Time: **40 minutes**

Servings **: 6**

Ingredients

- 3 ounces bacon
- 6 ounces brie cheese
- 1 chili pepper, seeded and chopped
- ¼ tsp parsley flakes
- **½ tsp paprika**

Directions

1. Set a pan over medium heat and fry the bacon until crispy; then crush it.
2. Place the other ingredients in a bowl and mix to combine with the bacon grease. Refrigerate the mixture for 20 minutes. Remove and form balls from the mixture.
3. **Set the bacon in a plate and roll the balls around to coat.**

Nutrition: Calories 456 - Total Fats 18g - Carbs: 41g - Protein 17g - Dietary Fiber: 1.8 g

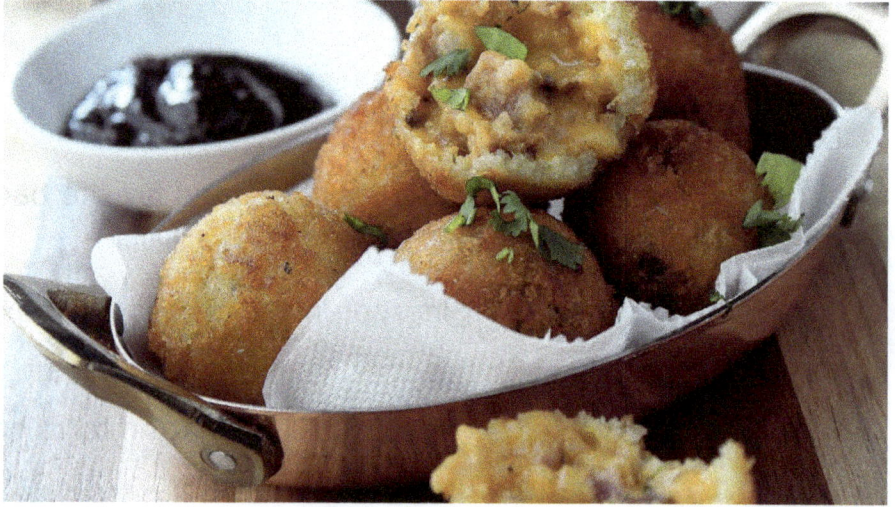

Creamy Cheddar Deviled Eggs

Preparation Time **: 10 minutes**

Cooking Time: **20 minutes**

Servings **: 6**

Ingredients

- 10 eggs
- ¼ cup mayonnaise
- 1 tbsp tomato paste
- 2 tbsp celery, chopped
- 2 tbsp carrot, chopped
- 2 tbsp chives, minced
- 2 tbsp cheddar cheese, grated
- **Salt and black pepper, to taste**

Directions

1. Place the eggs in a pot and fill with water by about 1 inch. Bring the eggs to a boil over high heat, then reduce the heat to medium and simmer for 10 minutes.

2. Remove and rinse under running water until cooled. Peel and discard the shell. Slice each egg in half lengthwise and get rid of the yolks.

3. **Mix the yolks with the rest of the ingredients. Split the mixture amongst the**

egg whites and set deviled eggs on a plate to serve.

Nutrition:

- Calories 156
- Fat 2.6 g
- Carbohydrates 1.5 g
- Sugar 0.1 g
- Protein 29 g
- Cholesterol 213 mg

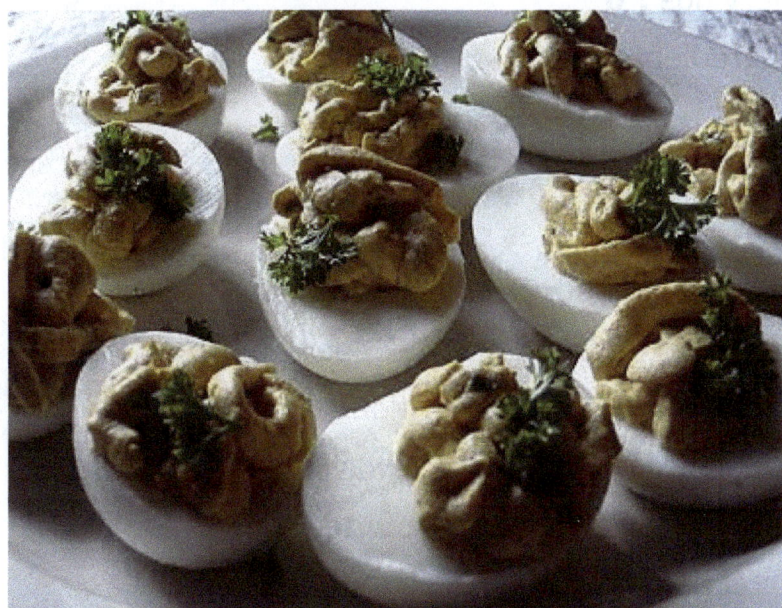

Jamon & Queso Balls

Preparation Time **: 10 minutes**

Cooking Time :30 minutes

Servings **: 6**

Ingredients

- 1 egg
- 6 slices jamon serrano, chopped
- 6 ounces cotija cheese
- 6 ounces Manchego cheese
- Salt and black pepper, to taste
- ¼ cup almond flour
- 1 tsp baking powder
- **1 tsp garlic powder**

Directions

1. Preheat oven to 420 °F.
2. Whisk the egg; place in the remaining ingredients and mix well. Split the mixture into 16 balls;
3. Set the balls on a baking sheet lined with parchment paper.
4. **Bake for 13 minutes or until they turn golden brown and become crispy.**

Nutrition:

- Calories 185
- Total Fats 8.5g
- Carbs: 0g
- Protein 27g
- Dietary Fiber: 0g

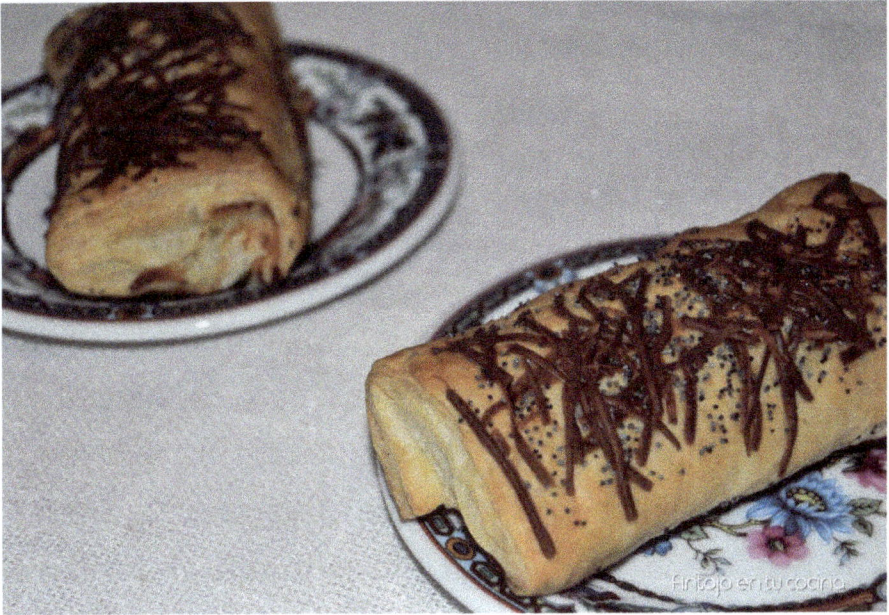

Cajun Crabmeat Frittata

Preparation Time : 10 minutes

Cooking Time: **20 minutes**

Servings **: 6**

Ingredients

- 1 tbsp olive oil
- 1 onion, chopped
- 4 ounces crabmeat, chopped
- 1 tsp cajun seasoning
- 6 large eggs, slightly beaten
- **½ cup Greek yogurt**

Directions

1. Preheat oven to 350ºF. Set a large skillet over medium heat and warm the oil. Add in onion and sauté until soft, about 3 minutes.
2. Stir in crabmeat and cook for 2 more minutes. Season with Cajun seasoning. Evenly distribute the ingredients at the bottom of the skillet.
3. **Whisk the eggs with yogurt. Transfer to the skillet. Set the skillet in the oven and bake for about 18 minutes or until eggs are cooked through. Slice into wedges and serve warm.**

Nutrition **:**

- Calories 280
- Total Fats 17g
- Carbs: 3g
- Protein 35g
- Dietary Fiber: 1g

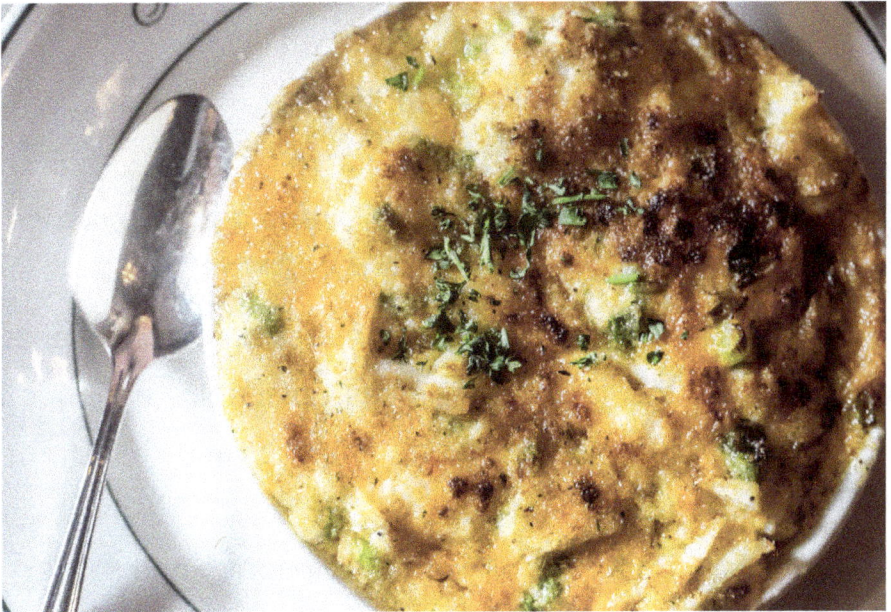

Crabmeat & Cheese Stuffed Avocado

Preparation Time: **10 minutes**

Cooking Time :50 minutes

Servings **: 6**

Ingredients

- 1 tsp olive oil
- 1 cup crabmeat
- 2 avocados, halved and pitted
- 3 ounces cream cheese
- ¼ cup almonds, chopped
- 1 tsp smoked paprika

Directions

1. Preheat oven to 425ºF and grease a baking pan with cooking spray.
2. In a bowl, mix crabmeat with cream cheese. To the avocado halves, place in almonds and crabmeat/cheese mixture and bake for 18 minutes.
3. Decorate with smoked paprika and serve.

Nutrition: Calories 300 - Total Fats 8g - Carbs: 5g - Protein 18g - Dietary Fiber: 2g

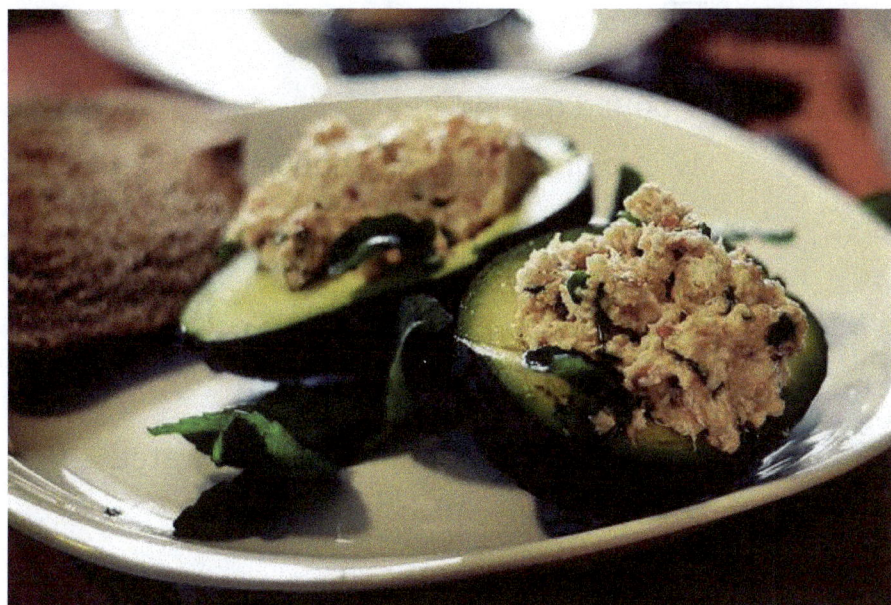

Juicy Beef Cheeseburgers

Preparation Time **: 10 minutes**

Cooking Time :20 minutes

Servings **: 6**

Ingredients

- 1 pound ground beef
- ½ cup green onions, chopped
- 2 garlic cloves, finely chopped
- ¼ tsp black pepper
- Salt and cayenne pepper, to taste
- 2 oz mascarpone cheese
- 3 oz pecorino Romano cheese, grated
- **2 tbsp olive oil**

Directions

1. In a mixing bowl, mix ground beef, garlic, cayenne pepper, black pepper, green onions, and salt. Shape into 6 balls; then flatten to make burgers.

2. In a separate bowl, mix mascarpone with grated pecorino Romano cheeses. Split the cheese mixture among prepared patties.

3. Wrap the meat mixture around the cheese mixture to ensure that the filling is sealed inside. Warm oil in a skillet over medium heat.

4. Cook the burgers for 5 minutes each side.

Nutrition:

- Calories 130
- Total Fats 8g
- Carbs: 5g
- Protein 16g
- Dietary Fiber: 2g

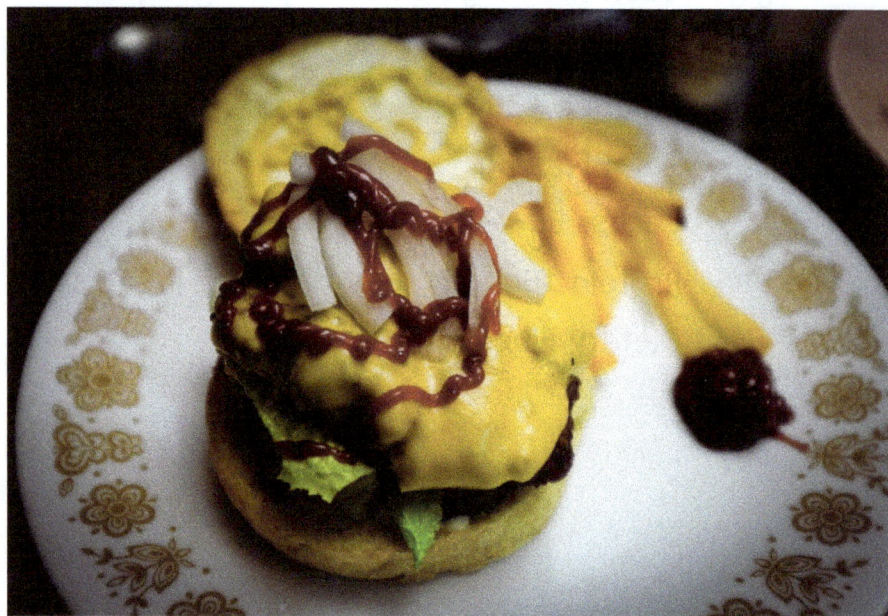

Cilantro & Chili Omelet
Preparation Time: 10 minutes

Cooking Time :20 minutes

Servings **: 6**

Ingredients

- 2 tsp butter
- 2 spring onions, chopped
- 2 spring garlic, chopped
- 4 eggs
- 1 cup sour cream, divided
- 2 tomatoes, sliced
- 1 green chili pepper, minced
- 2 tbsp fresh cilantro, chopped
- **Salt and black pepper, to taste**

Directions

1. Set a pan over high heat and warm the butter. Sauté garlic and onions until tender and translucent.
2. Whisk the eggs with sour cream. Pour into the pan and use a spatula to smooth the surface
3. Cooking until eggs become puffy and brown to bottom. Add cilantro, chili pepper and tomatoes to one side of the omelet.

4. Season with black pepper and salt. Fold the omelet in half and slice into wedges.

Nutrition:

- Calories – 216
- Fat – 4g
- Saturated Fat – 1g
- Trans Fat – 0g
- Carbohydrates – 2g
- Fiber – 0g
- Sodium – 346mg
- Protein – 8g

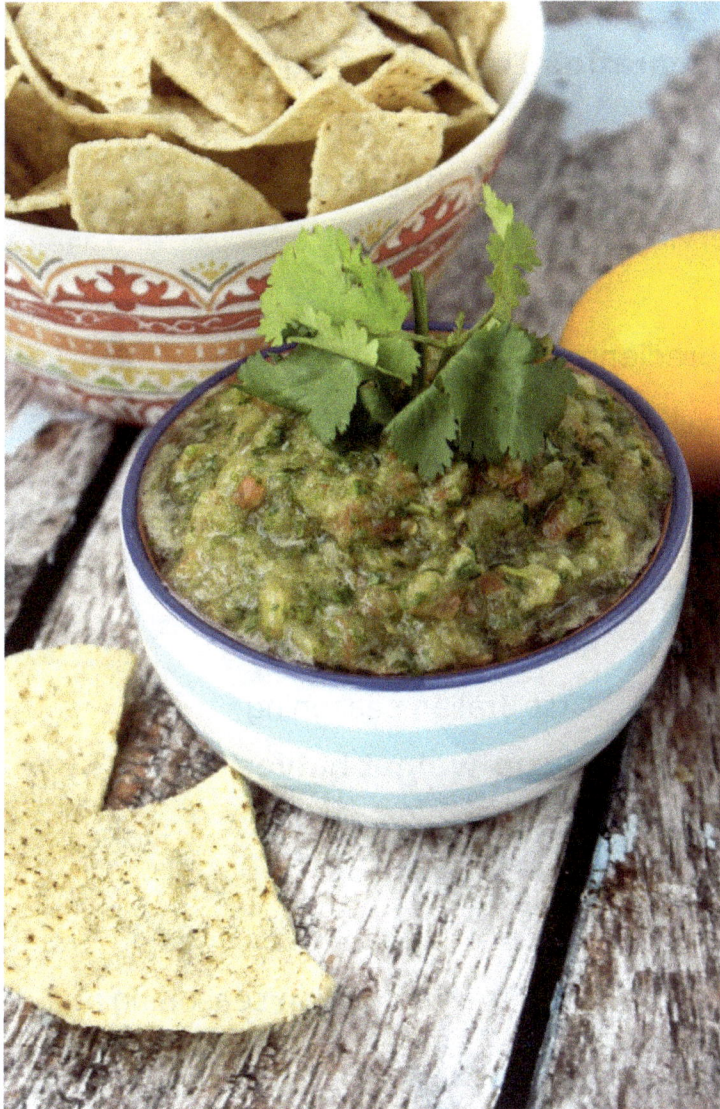

Zucchini with Blue Cheese and Walnuts

Preparation Time : 10 minutes

Cooking Time: **60 minutes**

Servings **: 6**

Ingredients

- 2 tbsp olive oil
- 6 zucchinis, sliced
- 1 ⅓ cups heavy cream
- 1 cup sour cream
- 8 ounces blue cheese
- 1 tsp Italian seasoning
- **¼ cup walnut halves**

Directions

1. Set a grill pan over medium heat. Season zucchinis with Italian seasoning and drizzle with olive oil. Grill the zucchini until lightly charred. Remove to a serving platter.
2. In a dry pan over medium heat, toast the walnuts for 2-3 minutes and set aside.

3. Add the heavy cream, blue cheese, and sour cream to the pan and mix until everything is well combined.
4. Let cool for a few minutes and scatter over the grilled zucchini. Top with walnuts to serve.

Nutrition:

- Calories 181
- Total Fats 11.5g
- Carbs: 1.8g
- Protein 27.3g
- Dietary Fiber: 0.7g

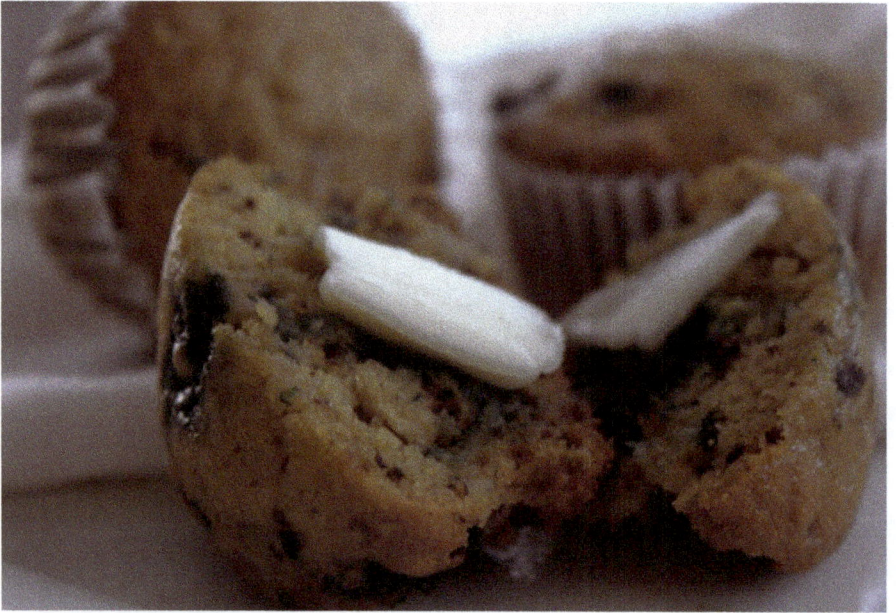

Garlick & Cheese Turkey Slices

Preparation Time: **10 minutes**

Cooking Time :20 minutes

Servings **: 6**

Ingredients

- 2 tbsp olive oil
- 1 pound turkey breasts, sliced
- 2 garlic cloves, minced
- ½ cup heavy cream
- ⅓ cup chicken broth
- 2 tbsp tomato paste
- **1 cup cheddar cheese, shredded**

Directions

1. Set a pan over medium heat and warm the oil; add in garlic and turkey and fry for 4 minutes; set aside.
2. Stir in the broth, tomato paste, and heavy cream Cooking until thickened.
3. Return the turkey to the pan; spread shredded cheddar cheese over.
4. **Let sit for 5 minutes covered or until the cheese melts. Serve instantly**

Nutrition:

- Calories 595
- Total Fats 31.5g
- Carbs: 52.6 g
- Protein 17.7g
- Dietary Fiber: 9.4g

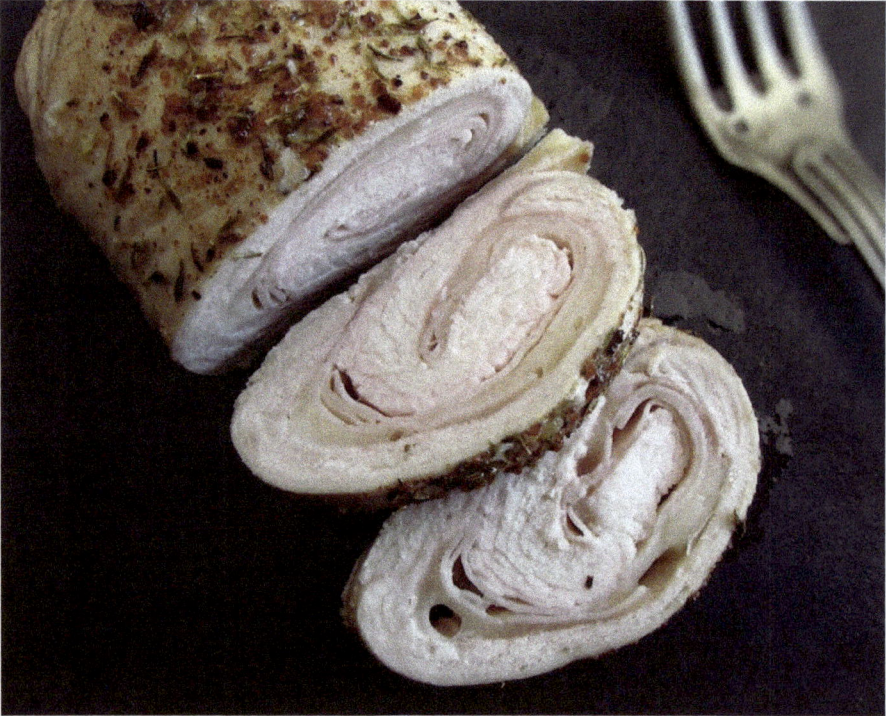

Prosciutto & Cheese Egg Cups

Preparation Time **: 10 minutes**

Cooking Time :60 minutes

Servings **: 6**

Ingredients

- 9 slices prosciutto
- 9 eggs
- 4 green onions, chopped
- ½ cup cheddar cheese, shredded
- ¼ tsp garlic powder
- ½ tsp dried dill weed
- Sea salt and black pepper, to taste

Directions

1. Preheat oven to 390ºF and grease a 9-cup muffin pan with oil.
2. Line one slice of prosciutto on each cup. In a mixing bowl, combine the remaining ingredients.
3. Split the egg mixture among muffin cups. Bake for 20 minutes.

Nutrition:

- Calories 221
- Fat 9.1 g

- Carbohydrates 12 g
- Sugar 0.3 g
- Protein 21.9 g
- Cholesterol 174 mg

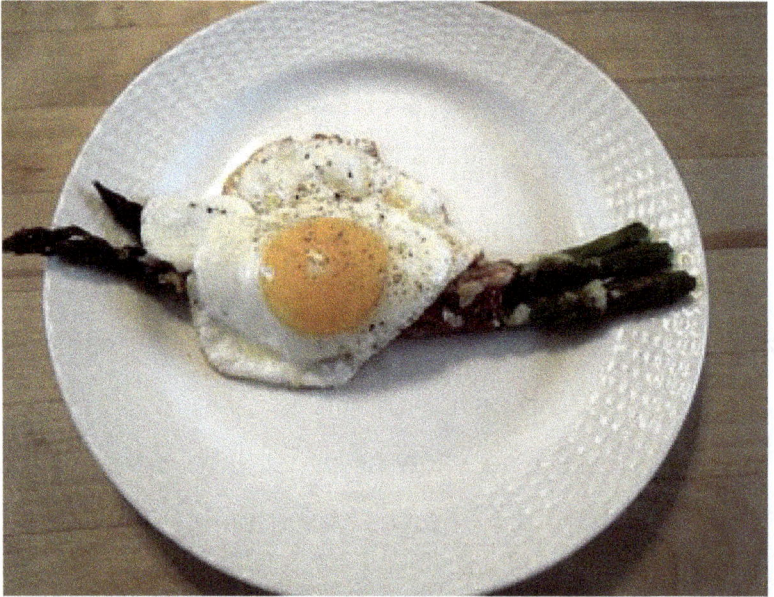

Spanish Salsa Aioli

Preparation Time: **10 minutes**

Cooking Time :20 minutes

Servings **: 6**

Ingredients

- 1 tbsp lemon juice
- 1 egg yolk, at room temperature
- 1 clove garlic, crushed
- ½ tsp salt
- ½ cup olive oil
- ¼ tsp black pepper
- **¼ cup fresh parsley, chopped**

Directions

1. Using a blender, place in salt, lemon juice, garlic, and egg yolk; pulse well to get a smooth and creamy mixture.
2. Set blender to slow speed.
3. Slowly sprinkle in olive oil and combine to ensure the oil incorporates well. Stir in parsley and black pepper.
4. **Refrigerate the mixture until ready.**

Nutrition:

- Calories 571

- Fat 35.1 g
- Carbohydrates 26 g
- Sugar 3.9 g
- Protein 36.9 g
- **Cholesterol 133 mg**

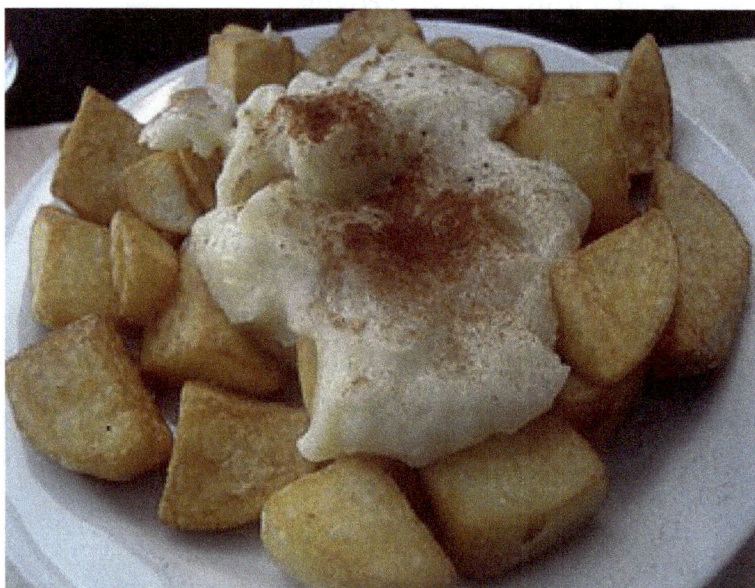

Three-Cheese Fondue with Walnuts and Parsley

Preparation Time: **10 minutes**

Cooking Time :50 minutes

Servings **: 6**

Ingredients

- ½ pound brie cheese, chopped
- ⅓ pound Swiss cheese, shredded
- ½ cup Emmental cheese, grated
- 1 tbsp xanthan gum
- ½ tsp garlic powder
- 1 tsp onion powder
- ¾ cup white wine
- ½ tbsp lemon juice
- Black pepper, to taste
- **1 cup walnuts, chopped**

Directions

1. Set broiler to preheat. In a skillet, thoroughly mix onion powder, brie, Emmental, Swiss cheese, garlic powder, and xanthan gum.
2. Pour in lemon juice and wine and sprinkle with black pepper.

3. **Set the skillet under the broiler for 6 to 7 minutes, until the cheese browns. Garnish with walnuts.**

Nutrition:

- Calories 290
- Fat 4.8 g
- Carbohydrates 40.1 g
- Sugar 5.2 g
- Protein 23.6 g
- Cholesterol 119 mg

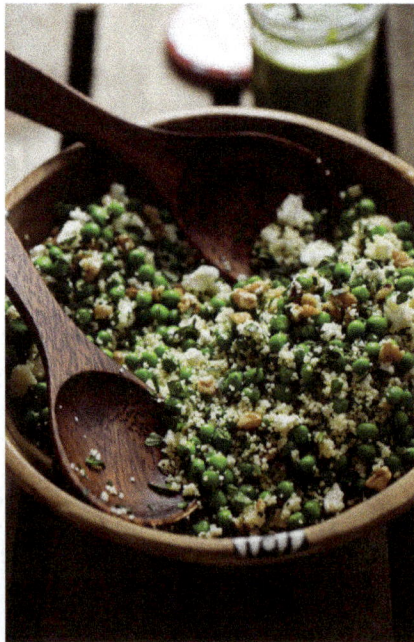

Mushroom Salad

Preparation Time: **10 minutes**

Cooking time: **10 minutes**

Servings **: 4**

Ingredients:

- 2 tablespoons butter
- 1 pound cremini mushrooms, chopped
- 2 tablespoons extra virgin olive oil
- Salt and ground black pepper, to taste
- 2 bunches arugula
- 4 slices prosciutto
- 2 tablespoons apple cider vinegar
- sundried tomatoes in oil, drained, and chopped
- Parmesan cheese, shaved
- **Fresh parsley leaves, chopped**

Directions:

1. Heat a pan with butter and half of the oil over medium–high heat.

2. Add mushrooms, salt, and pepper, stir, and cook for 3 minutes. Reduce heat, stir again, and cook for 3 more minutes.
3. Add rest of the oil and vinegar, stir and cook 1 minute.
4. Place arugula on a serving platter, add prosciutto on top, add the mushroom mixture, sundried tomatoes, more salt and pepper, Parmesan shavings, parsley, and serve.

Nutrition:

- Calories 211
- Fat 9.7 g
- Carbohydrates 1.7 g
- Sugar 0 g
- Protein 29.7 g
- Cholesterol 67 mg

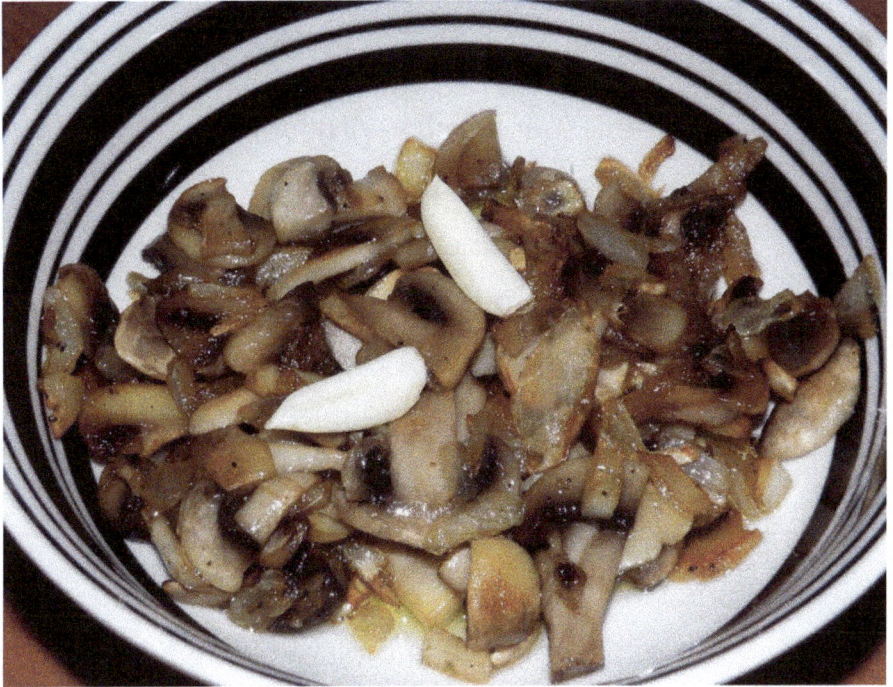

Greek Side Salad

Preparation Time: **10 minutes**

Cooking time : 7 minutes

Servings **: 4**

Ingredients:

- 1 and ½ pounds mushrooms, sliced
- 1 tablespoon extra-virgin olive oil
- 2 garlic cloves, peeled and minced
- 1 teaspoon dried basil
- Salt and ground black pepper, to taste
- 1 tomato, cored and diced
- 2 tablespoons lemon juice
- ½ cup water
- 1 tablespoons coriander, chopped

Directions :

1. Heat a pan with the oil over medium heat, add mushrooms, stir, and cook for 3 minutes.
2. Add basil and garlic, stir, and cook for 1 minute.
3. Add water, salt, pepper, tomato, and lemon juice, stir, and cook for a few minutes.
4. Take off heat, transfer to a bowl, set aside to cool down, sprinkle the coriander, and serve.

Nutrition:

- Calories 310
- Total Fats 13g
- Carbs: 10g
- Protein 40g
- Dietary Fiber: 3.5g

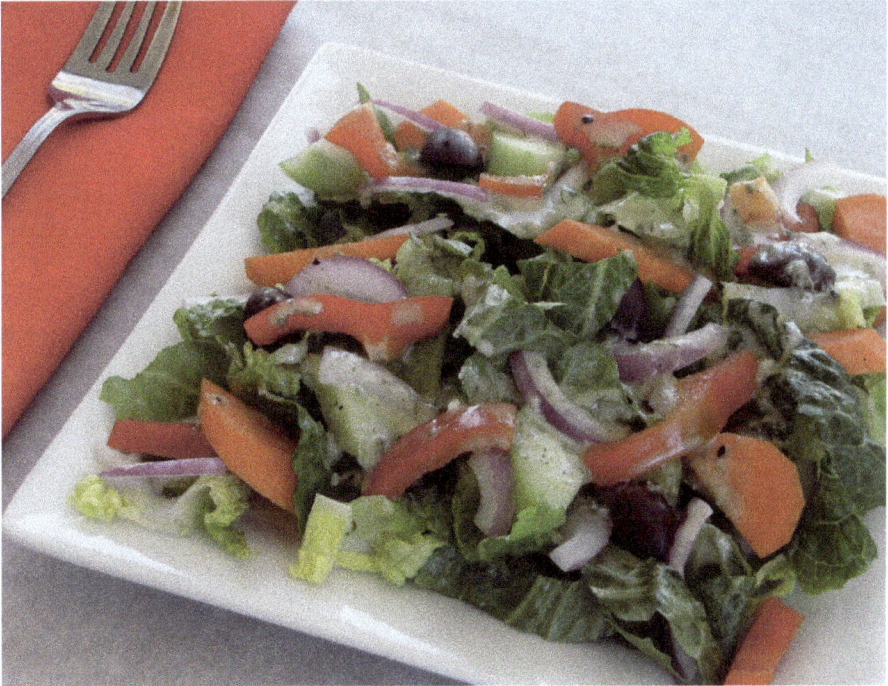

Tomato Salsa

Preparation Time **: 2 hours**

Servings: **4**

Ingredients **:**

- 3 yellow tomatoes, seeded and chopped
- 1 red tomato, seeded and chopped
- Salt and ground black pepper, to taste
- ⅓ cup onion, diced
- 1 jalapeño pepper, diced
- ¼ cup cilantro, diced
- 2 tablespoons lime juice
- 1/3 teaspoons stevia

Directions:

1. In a bowl, mix tomatoes with onion, and jalapeño.
2. Add cilantro, lime juice, salt, pepper, stevia, and stir well.
3. Cover the bowl, keep in the refrigerator for 2 hours, and serve.

Nutrition:

- Calories 150
- Total Fats 2g
- Carbs: 18g

- Protein 21g
- Dietary Fiber: 1g

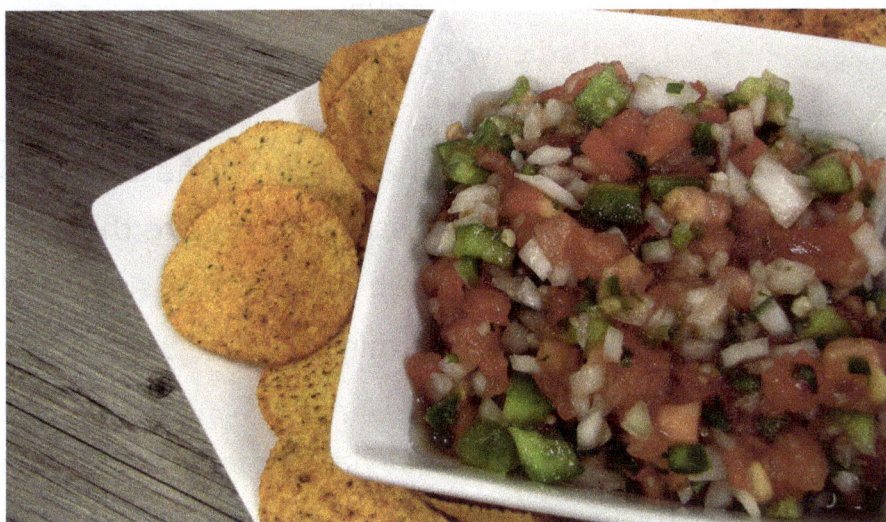

Grilled Steak Salad

Preparation and Cooking time **: 55 minutes**

Servings **: 4**

Ingredients **:**

- 1 Cucumber, sliced
- 1 cup Halved cherry tomatoes
- 1 package Mixed greens
- 1 lb. Flank steak
- Soy sesame dressing
- 1 Grated carrot

Directions **:**

1. Take out a bowl and add in the steak with a drizzle of the dressing. Make sure that all your steak is well coated with the dressing and then set aside for a minimum of 30 minutes to marinate.
2. After the steak has had some time to marinate, turn on the grill, and get it preheated to medium-high.
3. Remove the excess dressing and place the steak on the grill.
4. Let the steak grill until it reaches 145 degrees, which will take about 5 minutes on each side.

5. Move the steak to a plate and allow the steak to rest for at   least 5 minutes before slicing. Cutting the stake too soon will ruin the steak! Letting it rest is important to a juicy steak.
6. Plate your veggies first as the base of the bowl, then layer the steak over-top. Drizzle with some of the dressing and then serve.

Nutrition:

- Calories 192
- Total Fats 2g
- Carbs: 0.3gProtein 42gDietary Fiber: 0g

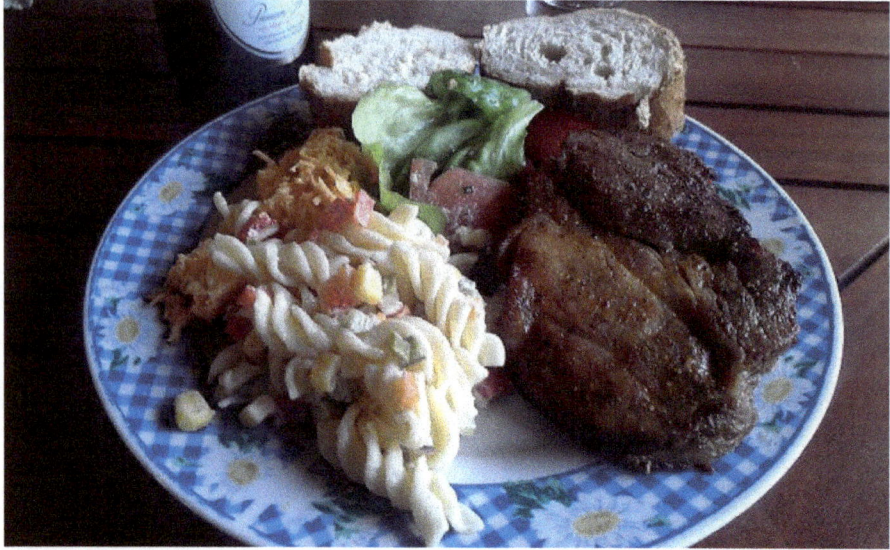

Feta & Sun-Dried Tomato Salad
Ingredients for 2 servings

5 sun-dried tomatoes in oil, sliced

3 oz bacon slices, chopped

4 basil leaves

1 cup feta cheese, crumbled

2 tsp extra virgin olive oil

1 tsp balsamic vinegar

Salt to taste

Directions and Total Time: approx. 10 minutes

Fry the bacon in a pan over medium heat, until golden and crisp, about 5 minutes. Remove with a perforated spoon and set aside. Arrange the sun-dried tomatoes on a serving plate. Scatter feta cheese over and top with basil leaves. Add the crispy bacon on top, drizzle with olive oil and sprinkle with vinegar and salt.

Per serving: Cal 411; Fat 36g; Net Carbs 2.5g; Protein 16g

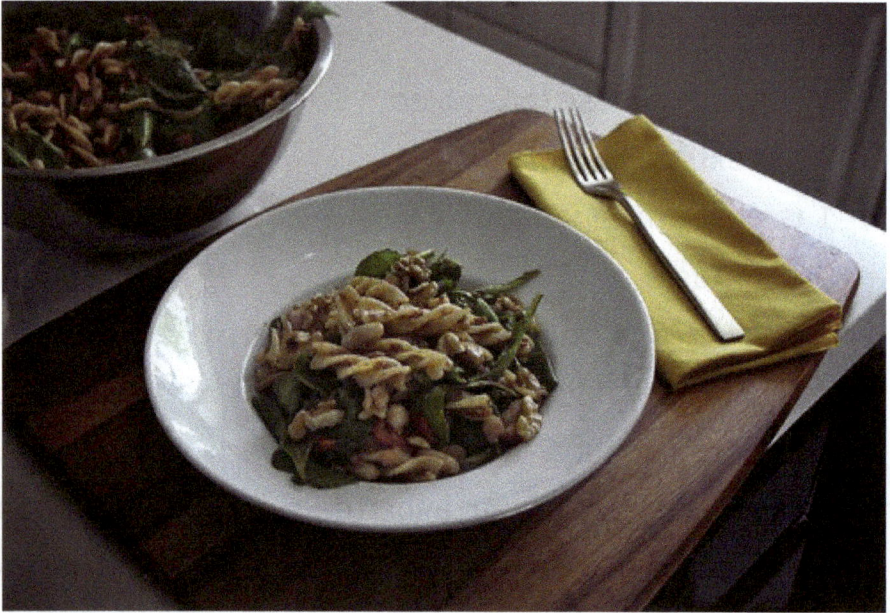

Cobb Salad with Roquefort Dressing

<u>Ingredients</u> for 4 servings

½ cup Roquefort cheese, crumbled

½ cup whipping cream

¼ cup buttermilk

½ cup mayonnaise

1 tbsp Worcestershire sauce

1 tbsp chives, chopped

3 eggs, hard-boiled, chopped

1 chicken breast

4 oz bacon, cooked, crumbled

1 cup endive, chopped

½ romaine lettuce, chopped

1 cup watercress

1 avocado, pitted and diced

1 large tomato, chopped

½ cup feta cheese, crumbled

Salt and black pepper to taste

<u>Directions</u> and Total Time: approx. 20 minutes

In a bowl, whisk the whipping cream, buttermilk, mayonnaise, and Worcestershire sauce. Stir in the

Roquefort cheese, salt, pepper, and chives. Keep in the fridge.

Preheat the grill pan over high heat. Season the chicken with salt and pepper. Grill for 3 minutes on each side. Remove to a plate to cool for 3 minutes, and cut into bite-size chunks. Place the lettuce, endive, and watercress on a salad bowl and add the avocado, tomato, eggs, bacon, and chicken. Sprinkle the feta cheese over the salad and drizzle with the cheese dressing.

Per serving: Cal 527; Fat 43g; Net Carbs 7.2g; Protein 28g

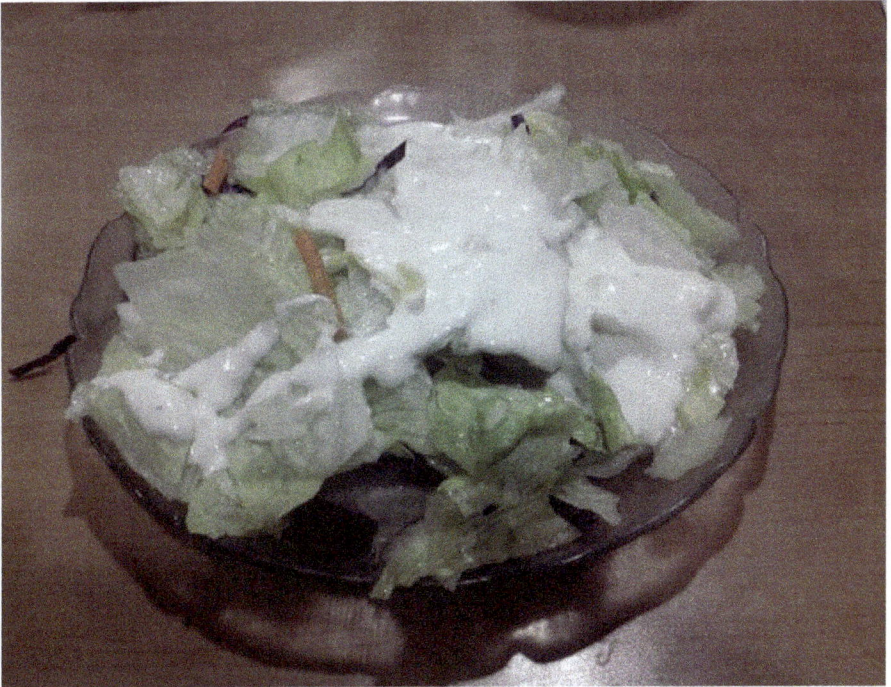

Pesto Caprese Salad with Tuna

Ingredients for 2 servings

4 oz canned tuna chunks in water, drained

1 tomato, sliced

1 ball fresh mozzarella, sliced

4 basil leaves

½ cup pine nuts

½ cup Parmesan, grated

½ cup extra virgin olive oil

½ lemon, juiced

Directions and Total Time: approx. 10 minutes

Put in a food processor the basil leaves, pine nuts, Parmesan cheese, and extra virgin olive oil, and blend until smooth. Stir in the lemon juice. Arrange the cheese and tomato slices on a serving plate. Scatter the tuna chunks and pesto over the top and serve.

Per serving: Cal 364; Fat 31g; Net Carbs 1g; Protein 21g

Sausage & Pesto Salad with Cheese
Ingredients for 2 servings

½ cup mixed cherry tomatoes, cut in half

½ lb pork sausage links, sliced

1 cups mixed lettuce greens

¼ cup radicchio, sliced

1 tbsp olive oil

¼ lb feta cheese, cubed

½ tbsp lemon juice

¼ cup basil pesto

6 black olives, pitted, halved

Salt and black pepper, to taste

1 tbsp Parmesan shavings

Directions and Total Time: approx. 10 minutes

Cook the sausages in warm olive oil over medium heat for 5-6 minutes, stirring often. In a salad bowl, combine the mixed lettuce greens, radicchio, feta cheese, pesto, cherry tomatoes, black olives, and lemon juice and toss well to coat. Season with salt and black pepper and add the sausages. Sprinkle with Parmesan shavings and serve.

Per serving: Cal 611; Fat 48g; Net Carbs 7.5g; Protein 31g

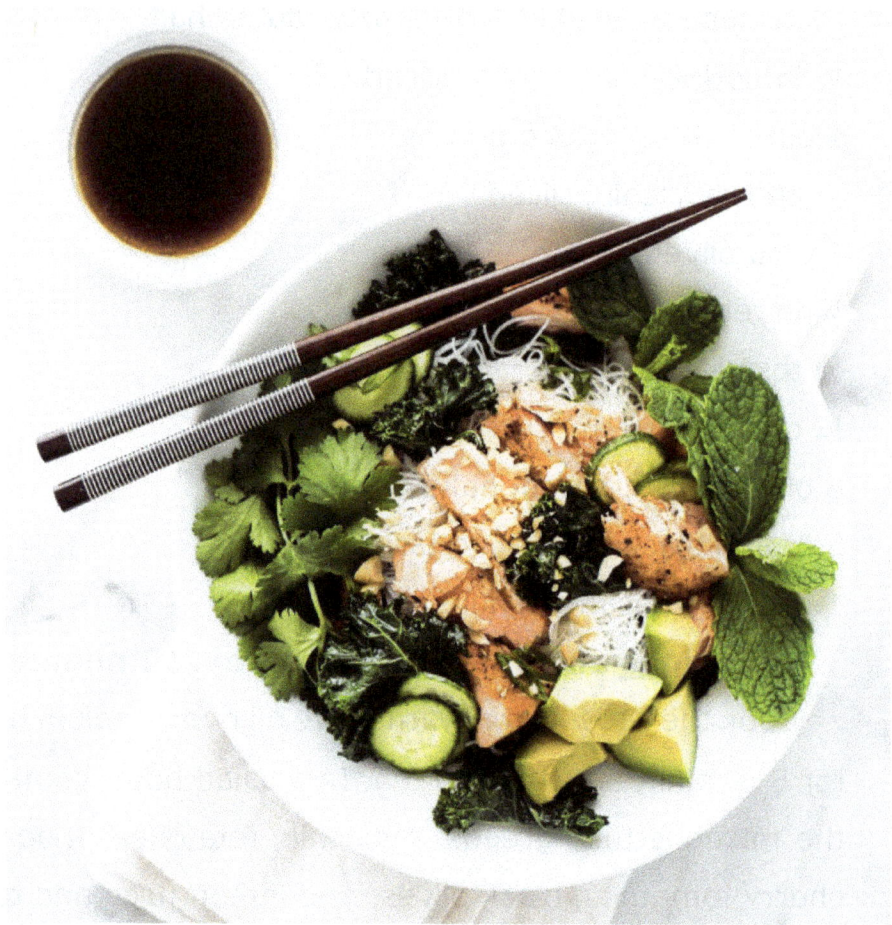

Smoked Salmon, Bacon & Egg Salad

<u>Ingredients</u> for 4 servings

2 eggs

1 head romaine lettuce, torn

4 oz smoked salmon, chopped

3 slices bacon

4 cherry tomatoes, halved

Salt and black pepper to taste

Dressing:

½ cup mayonnaise

½ tsp garlic puree

1 tbsp lemon juice

1 tsp tabasco sauce

<u>Directions</u> and Total Time: approx. 20 minutes

In a bowl, mix well the dressing ingredients and set aside. Bring a pot of salted water to a boil. Crack each egg into a small bowl and gently slide into the water. Poach for 2-3 minutes. Remove with a perforated spoon, transfer to a paper towel to dry, and plate. Put the bacon in a skillet over medium heat and fry until browned and crispy, about 6 minutes, turning once. Remove, allow cooling, and chop into small pieces. Toss the lettuce, smoked salmon, bacon, and dressing in a salad bowl.

Divide the salad between plates, top with the eggs each, and serve immediately or chilled.

Per serving: Cal 291; Fat 19g; Net Carbs 6.4g; Protein 15g

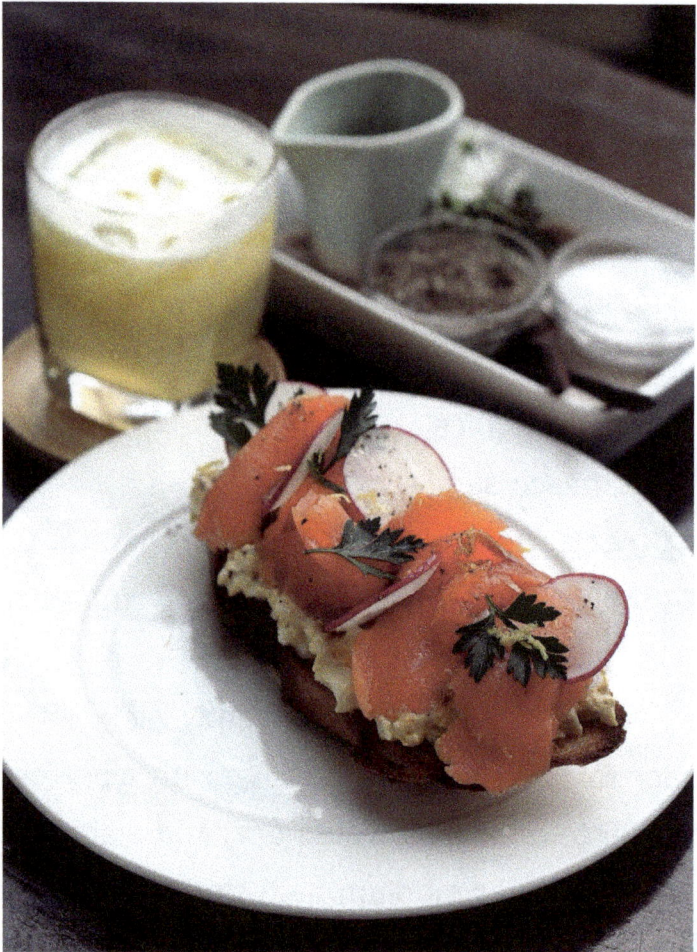

Classic Egg Salad with Olives

Ingredients for 2 servings

4 eggs

¼ cup mayonnaise

½ tsp sriracha sauce

½ tbsp mustard

¼ cup scallions

¼ stalk celery, minced

Salt and black pepper, to taste

1 head romaine lettuce, torn

¼ tsp fresh lime juice

10 black olives

Directions and Total Time: approx. 15 minutes

Boil the eggs in salted water over medium heat for 10 minutes. When cooled, peel and chop them into bite-size pieces. Place in a salad bowl. Stir in the remaining ingredients, except for the scallions, until everything is well combined. Scatter the scallions all over and decorate with black olives to serve.

Per serving: Cal 312; Fat 22g; Net Carbs 6.3g; Protein 17g

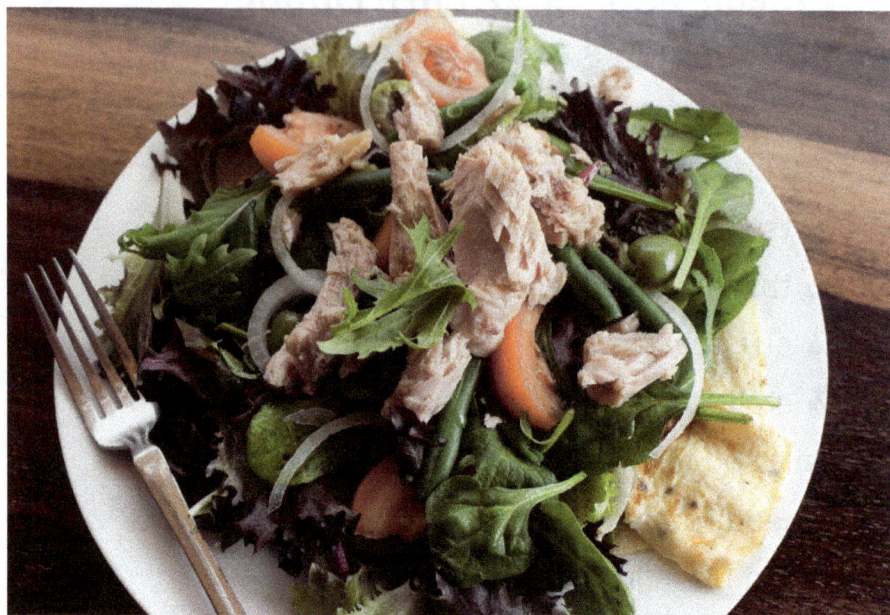

Broccoli and Turkey Dish

Preparation time **: 5 minutes** Cooking time: **15 minutes**

Servings **: 6**

Ingredients

- ¼ tsp red pepper flakes
- 1 tbsp olive oil
- 1 tsp soy sauce
- 4 oz broccoli florets
- 4 oz cauliflower florets, riced
- **4 oz ground turkey**

Directions

1. Bring out a skillet pan, place it over medium heat, add olive oil and when hot, add beef, crumble it and cook for 8 minutes until no longer pink.

2. **Then add broccoli florets and riced cauliflower, stir well, drizzle with soy sauce and sesame oil, season with salt, black pepper, and red pepper flakes and continue cooking for 5 minutes until vegetables have thoroughly cooked.**

Nutrition:

- Calories – 263 Fat – 14g

- Saturated Fat – 2g
- Trans Fat – 0g
- Carbohydrates – 36g
- Fiber – 11g
- Sodium – 168mg
- Protein – 5g

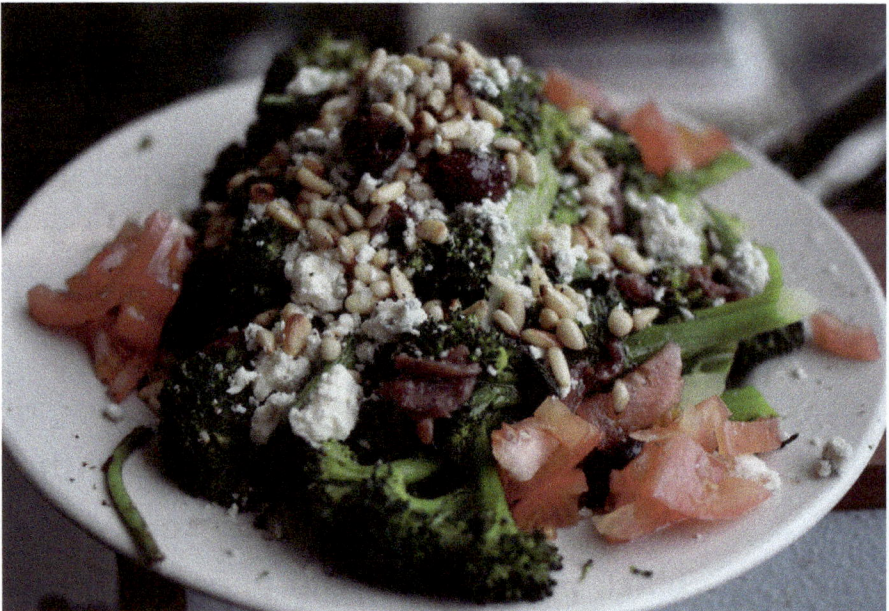

Easy Mayo Salmon

Preparation time : 5 minutes Cooking time: 10 minutes

Servings : 6

Ingredients

- 2 salmon fillets
- 4 tbsp mayonnaise

Directions

1. Turn on the Panini press, spray it with oil and let it preheat.
2. Then spread 1 tbsp of mayonnaise on each side of salmon, place them on Panini press pan, shut with lid, and cook for 7 to 10 minutes until salmon has cooked to the desired level.

Nutrition

- Calories - 203
- Fat – 7g
- Carbohydrates – 33g
- Fiber – 2g
- Protein – 4.5g

Zesty Avocado and Lettuce Salad

Preparation time: 5 minutes Cooking time : 0 minutes

Servings : 6

Ingredients

- ½ of a lime, juiced
- 1 avocado, pitted, sliced
- 2 tbsp olive oil
- 4 oz chopped lettuce
- 4 tbsp chopped chives

Directions

1. Prepare the dressing and for this, bring out a small bowl, add oil, lime juice, salt, and black pepper, stir until mixed, and then slowly mix oil until combined.
2. Bring out a large bowl, add avocado, lettuce, and chives, and then toss gently.
3. Drizzle with dressing, toss until well coated, and then serve.

Nutrition: Calories 170 - Fat: 13.8g - Carbo: 3.4g - Dietary Fiber: 1.4g - Protein: 9.7g

Veggie, Bacon and Egg Dish

Preparation time **: 5 minutes** Cooking time **: 5 minutes**

Servings **: 6**

Ingredients

- ¼ cup mayonnaise
- 2 eggs, boiled, sliced
- 4 oz spinach
- **4 slices of bacon, chopped**

Directions

1. Bring out a skillet pan, place it over medium heat, add bacon, and cook for 5 minutes until browned.
2. In the meantime, bring out a salad bowl, add spinach in it, top with bacon and eggs and drizzle with mayonnaise.
3. **Toss until well mixed and then serve.**

Nutrition: Calories 63 - Fat: 4.4g - Carbohydrates: 0.3g - Dietary Fiber: 0g - Protein: 5.5g

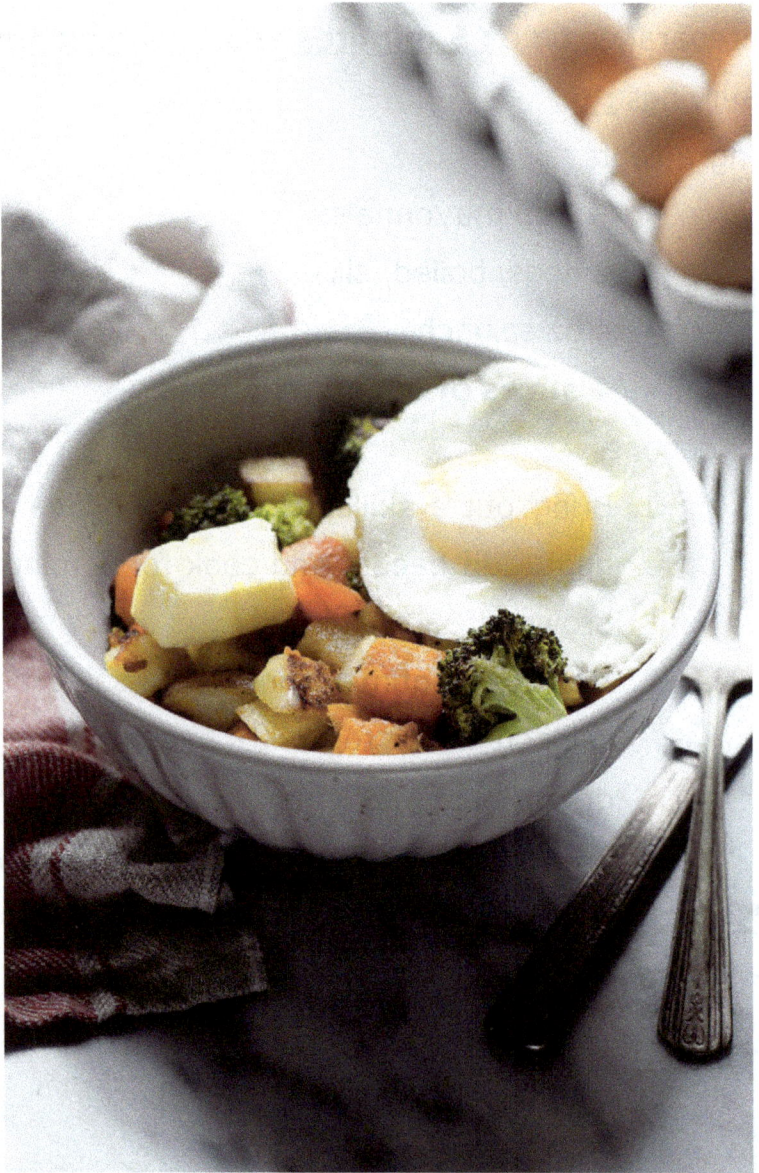

Keto Teriyaki Chicken

Preparation time: **5 minutes** Cooking time **: 18 minutes**
Servings **: 6**

Ingredients

- 1 tbsp olive oil
- 1 tbsp swerve sweetener
- 2 chicken thighs, boneless
- **2 tbsp soy sauce**

Directions

1. Bring out a skillet pan, place it over medium heat, add oil and when hot, add chicken thighs and cook for 5 minutes per side until seared.
2. Then sprinkle sugar over chicken thighs, drizzle with soy sauce and bring the sauce to boil.
3. Switch heat to medium-low level, continue cooking for 3 minutes until chicken is evenly glazed, and then transfer to a plate.
4. **Serve chicken with cauliflower rice.**

Nutrition : Calories 471 - Fat: 31.7g - Carbo: 4.3g - Dietary Fiber: 1.3g - Protein: 42.9g

Low Carb Keto Pasta and Tomato Sauce

Preparation time **: 40 minutes** Cooking time: **7 minute
s**

Servings **: 6**

Ingredients

- ¼ tsp ground black pepper
- ¼ tsp salt
- 2 egg yolks
- 2 tbsp tomato sauce
- **4 oz grated mozzarella cheese**

Directions

1. Bring out a heatproof bowl, add mozzarella in it, and microwave for 2 minutes or until it melts.

2. Whisk in yolks until combined, bring out a baking dish lined with parchment paper, and add cheese mixture in it.

3. Cover the cheese mixture with another parchment paper, press and spread the cheese mixture as thinly as possible, let it rest for 10 minutes until slightly firm.

4. Then uncover it, cut out thin spaghetti by using a knife and refrigerate the pasta for 45 minutes.
5. When ready to cook, bring out a saucepan half full of salty water, bring it to boil, add pasta and cook for 5 minutes until spaghetti is tender.
6. Drain the spaghetti, distribute it between two bowls, top with tomato sauce, season with salt and black pepper, toss until well mixed, and then serve.

Nutrition :

- Calories 641
- Fat: 15g
- Carbohydrates 16.4g
- Fiber 6g
- Protein 14.43g

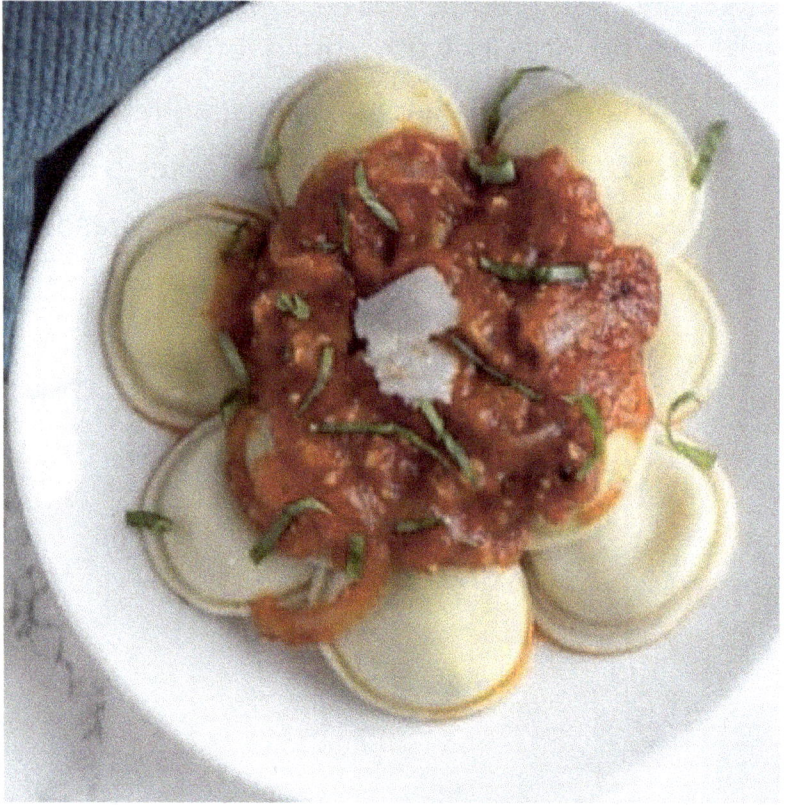

Lemon Garlic Shrimp Pasta

Preparation Time **: 10 minutes**

Cooking Time: **15 minutes**

Servings **: 4**

Ingredients:

- Linguine pasta (2 bags)
- Garlic cloves (4)
- Olive oil (2 tbsp.)
- Butter (2 tbsp.)
- Lemon (.5 of 1)
- Large raw shrimp (1 lb.)
- Paprika (.5 tsp.)
- Fresh basil (as desired)
- **Pepper and salt (as desired)**

Directions:

1. Drain the water from the package of noodles and rinse them in cold water. Add them to a pot of boiling water for two minutes. Transfer to a hot skillet over medium heat to remove the excess liquid (dry roast). Set them aside.

2. Use the same pan to warm the butter, oil, and mashed garlic. Sauté for a few minutes, but don't brown.

3. Slice the lemon into rounds and add them to the garlic along with the shrimp. Sauté for approximately three minutes per side.

4. **Add the noodles and spices and stir to blend the flavors.**

Nutrition:

- Calories 281.93
- Fat 29.14g
- Carbohydrates 6.76g
- Fiber 2.04
- **Protein 2.83g**

Easy Spicy Beans

Preparation time: **5 minutes** Cooking time **: 10 minutes**

Servings **: 6**

Ingredients

- ¼ tsp crushed red pepper
- ½ tsp minced garlic
- 1 ½ tbsp olive oil
- **4 oz green beans**

Directions

1. Bring out a saucepan half full of salted water, place it over medium heat, bring the water to boil, then add green beans and cook for 4 minutes until tender.
2. Drain the beans, wipe the pan, return it over medium heat, add oil and when hot, add garlic and cook for 1 minute until fragrant.
3. Then add green beans, season with salt and black pepper, cook for 1 minute and transfer beans to a plate.
4. Sprinkle red pepper on the green beans and serve.

Lime Chicken with Coleslaw

Preparation time: <u>35 minutes</u> **Cooking time:** <u>8 minutes</u> **Servings** : <u>6</u>

Ingredients

- ¼ tsp minced garlic
- ½ of a lime, juiced, zested
- ¾ tbsp apple cider vinegar
- 1 chicken thigh, boneless
- **2 oz coleslaw**

Directions

1. Prepare the marinade and for this, bring out a medium bowl, add vinegar, oil, garlic, paprika, salt, lime juice, and zest and stir until well mixed.

2. Cut chicken thighs into bite-size pieces, toss until well mixed, and marinate it in the refrigerator for 30 minutes.

3. Then Bring out a skillet pan, place it over medium-high heat, add butter and marinated chicken pieces and cook for 8 minutes until golden brown and thoroughly cooked.

4. **Serve chicken with coleslaw.**

Nutrition:

- Calories 400 Total Fats 30g

- Carbs: 9g Protein 20g
- Dietary Fiber: 0.8g

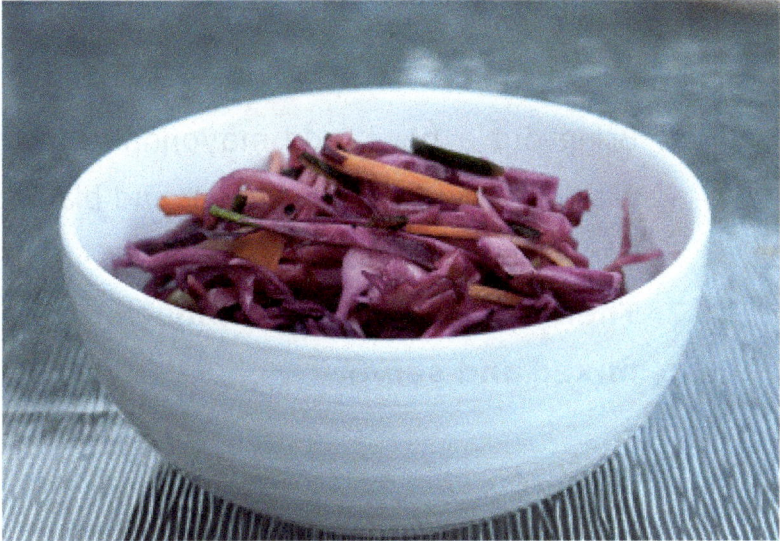

Spinach and Tuna Salad

Preparation time **: 5 minutes** Cooking time: **0 minutes**

Servings **: 6**

Ingredients

- 1 tbsp grated mozzarella cheese
- 1/3 cup mayonnaise
- 2 oz chopped spinach
- 4 oz tuna, packed in water

Directions

1. Bring out a bowl, add mayonnaise in it along with cheese, season with salt and black pepper and whisk until combined.

2. **Then add tuna and spinach, toss until mixed and serve.**

Nutrition:

- Calories 337
- Fat 18.1 g
- Carbohydrates 40.3 g
- Sugar 13.7 g
- Protein 6.4 g
- Cholesterol 0 mg

Sautéed Sausage and Beans

Preparation time **: 5 minutes** Cooking time **: 4 minutes**

Servings **: 6**

Ingredients

- ¼ tsp dried oregano
- 1 cup of water
- 1 tbsp olive oil
- 4 oz chicken sausage, sliced
- **4 oz green beans**

Directions

1. Turn on the instant pot, place all the ingredients in the inner pot, stir and shut with lid.
2. Press the manual button, cook for 4 minutes at high-pressure setting, and, when done, do quick pressure release.

Grilled Chicken with Spinach and Mozzarella

Preparation Time: **20 minutes** Cooking Time: **40 minutes** Servings **: 6**

Ingredients:

- Large chicken breasts (24 oz. or 6 portions)
- Olive oil (1 tsp.)
- Pepper and Kosher salt (as desired)
- Garlic cloves (3 crushed)
- Drained frozen spinach (10 oz.)
- Roasted red pepper strips packed in water (.5 cup)
- Shredded part-skim mozzarella (3 oz.)
- **Olive oil cooking spray**

Directions:

1. Warm the oven to 400º Fahrenheit.
2. Prepare the grill/grill pan with the oil.
3. Sprinkle the salt and pepper onto the chicken. Cook about two to three minutes per side.
4. Add the oil into a frying pan along with the garlic. Continue cooking for about 30 seconds, add a sprinkle of salt and pepper, and toss in

the spinach. Sauté another two to three minutes.

5. Arrange the chicken on a baking sheet and add the spinach to each one. Top them off with half of the cheese and peppers. Bake for about three minutes until lightly toasted.

6. Serve.

Nutrition:

- Calories 392 Fat 29 g
- Carbohydrates 32.6 g Sugar 13.7 g
- Protein 4.6 g Cholesterol 1 mg

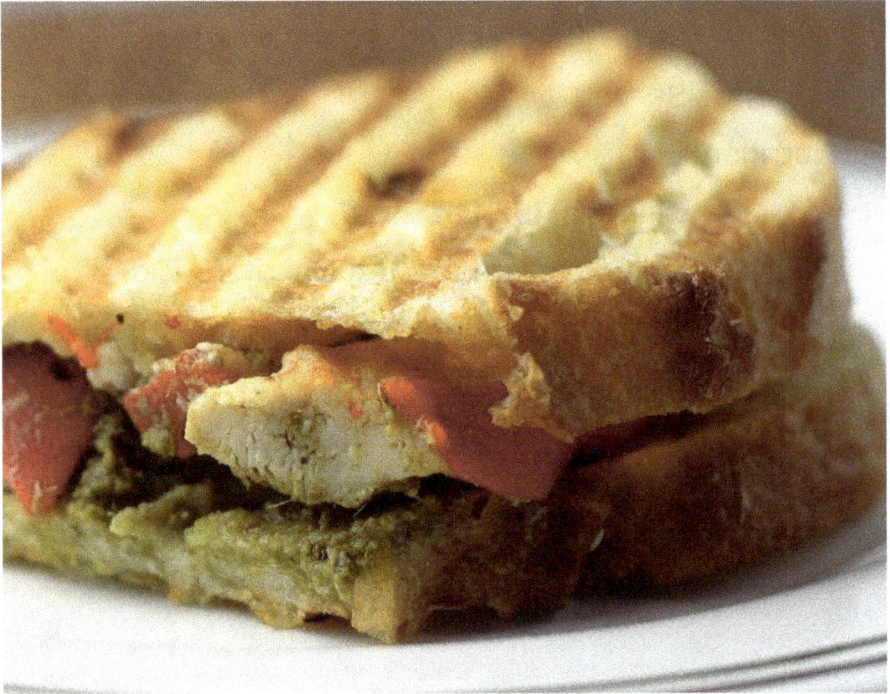

Cheese and Bacon Stuffed Zucchini

Preparation time **: 5 minutes** Cooking time **: 20 minutes**

Servings **: 6**

Ingredients

- 1 tbsp chopped spinach
- 1 tbsp grated mozzarella cheese
- 1 zucchini, halved lengthwise
- 2 slices of bacon
- **3 tbsp cream cheese**

Directions

1. Turn on the oven, then set it to 350 degrees F and let it preheat.
2. In the meantime, cut zucchini into half lengthwise, then use a spoon to remove the seedy center and set aside until required.
3. Place remaining ingredients, except for bacon in a bowl, stir well, and then evenly stuffed this mixture into zucchini.

4. **Wrap each zucchini half with a bacon slice, place them on a baking sheet lined with parchment paper and cook for 15 to 20 minutes until zucchini is tender and bacon is browned.**

Nutrition:

- Calories 255
- Fat 5 g
- Carbohydrates 44.9 g
- Sugar 17.1 g
- Protein 9.2 g
- **Cholesterol 9 mg**

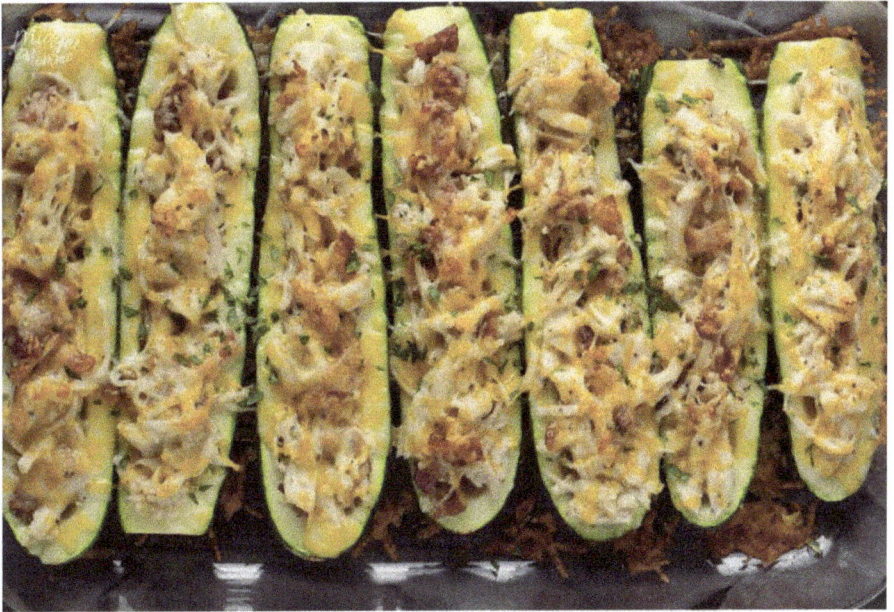

Chicken and Greens Soup

Preparation Time: **12 minutes**

Cooking Time :1 hour 50 minutes

Servings **: 8**

Ingredients **:**

- 1/4 cup of olive oil
- 1 1/2 lbs. chicken breast, boneless, cut into cube
- 1 spring onion, cut into cubes
- 1 clove of garlic, finely chopped
- 1 1/2 lettuce cos or romain, chopped
- 1 cup of fresh spinach finely chopped
- 1 bunch of dill finely chopped, without the thick stalks
- 1/2 Tablespoon of sweet chill powder
- 1 teaspoon of fresh mint, chopped
- 1 teaspoon of fresh thyme, chopped
- Salt and freshly ground pepper
- **5 cups of water**

Directions **:**

1. In a deep pot, heat the olive oil to a high heat and sauté the chicken for about 5 - 6 minutes.

2. Add the onion and sauté for about 3 minutes until softened.
3. Add the garlic, the lettuce, spinach, dill, mint, thyme and sauté for about 3-4 minutes, stirring with a wooden spoon.
4. Sprinkle with chili, salt, freshly ground pepper and pour 5 cups of water.
5. Bring to boil and cook for 1 1/2 hours on low heat.
6. **Serve hot.**

Nutrition:

- Calories: 122
- Carbohydrates: 11.5g
- Protein: 5.1g
- Fat: 8g
- Sugar: 2.8g
- Sodium: 69mg

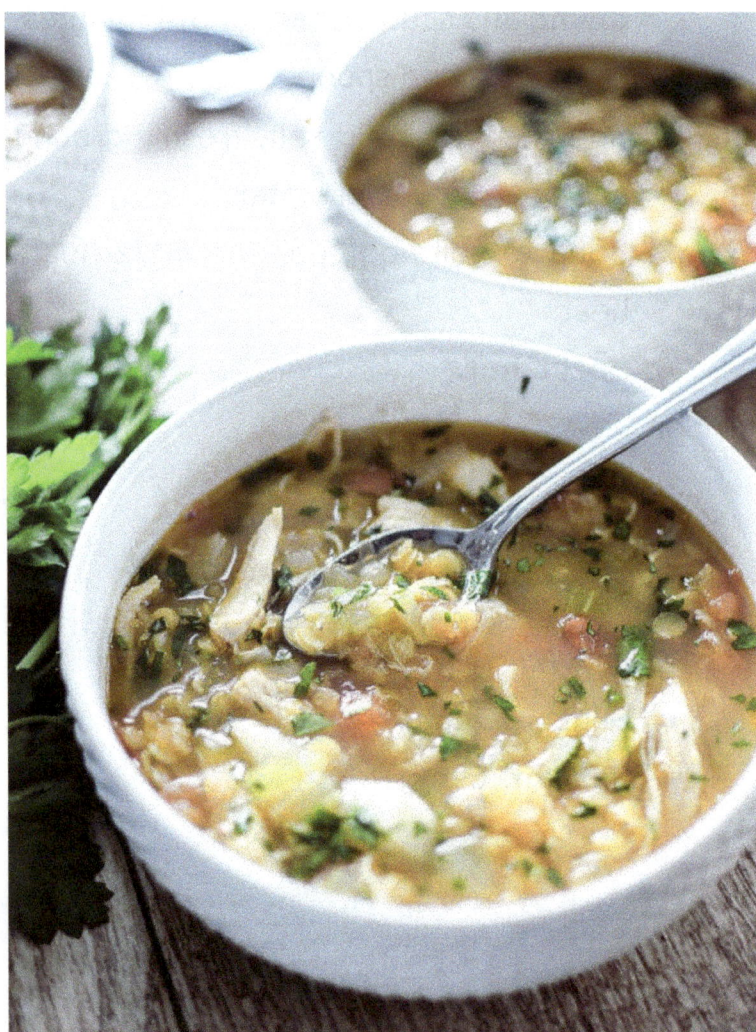

Cold Cauliflower and Cilantro Soup

Preparation Time **: 5 minutes**

Cooking Time :25 minutes

Servings **: 8**

Ingredients **:**

- 1 1/2 lbs. cauliflower previously steamed
- 1 cup almond milk
- 1/2 teaspoon fresh ginger grated
- 2 bunches fresh cilantro
- Tablespoon garlic-infused olive oil
- **pinch of salt**

Directions **:**

1. Heat water in a large pot until boiling. Place the steamer in a pot and put in the cauliflower.
2. Cover and steam cauliflower for 6 - 7 minutes.

3. Remove the cauliflower along with all ingredients from the list above in a high-speed blender.
4. Blend until smooth or until desired texture is achieved.
5. Pour the soup in a glass container, cover and refrigerate for 2 - 3 hours.
6. **Serve cold.**

Nutrition:

- Calories: 293
- Carbohydrates: 24.7g
- Protein: 3.8g
- Fat: 21.2g
- Sugar: 2.9g
- **Sodium: 223mg**

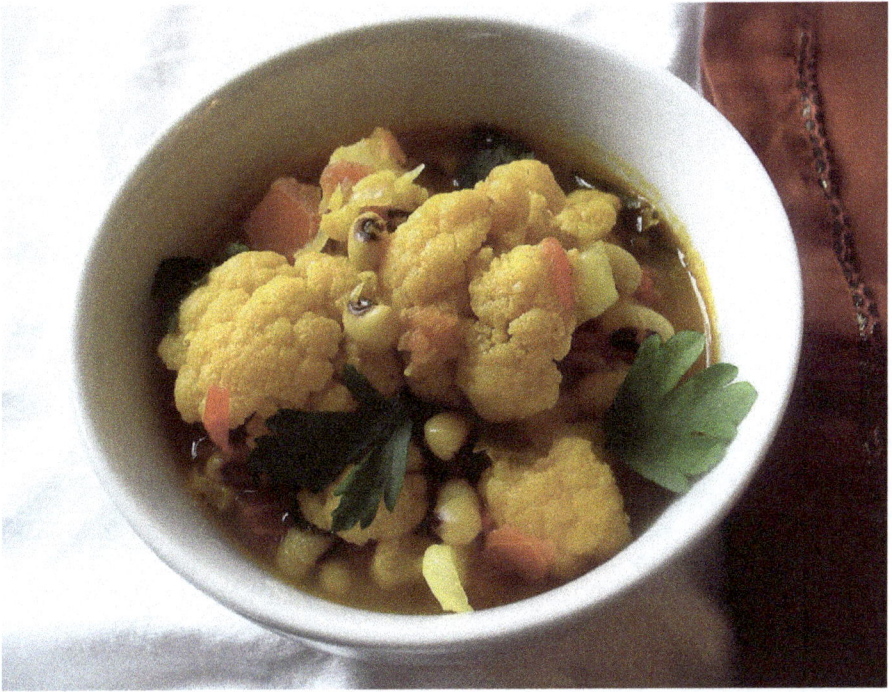

Creamy Broccoli Soup with Nutmeg

Preparation Time: **15 minute s**

Cooking Time :20 minutes

Servings **: 8**

Ingredients **:**

- Tablespoon of olive oil
- 2 green onions finely chopped
- 1 lb. broccoli floret, frozen or fresh
- 1 cups of bone broth cold
- 1 cup of cream
- Salt and ground pepper to taste
- **1 Tablespoon of nutmeg**

Directions **:**

1. Heat the olive oil in a pot over medium-high heat.
2. Add the onion in and sauté it until becomes translucent.
3. Add the broccoli, season with the salt and pepper, and bring to boil.
4. Cover the pot and cook for 6 - 8 minutes.
5. Transfer the broccoli mixture into blender, and blend until smooth.

6. Pour the cream, and blend for further 30 seconds.

7. Return the soup in a pot and reheat it.

8. **Adjust salt and pepper and serve hot with grated nutmeg.**

Nutrition:

- Calories 165
- Fat 2.8 g
- Carbohydrates 30.9 g
- Sugar 13.6 g
- Protein 5.3 g
- **Cholesterol 5 mg**

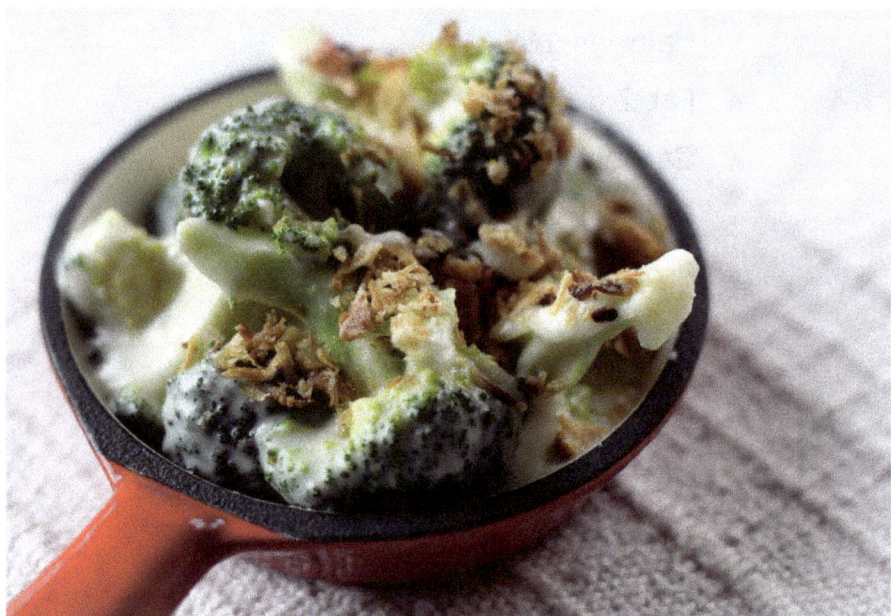

Creamy Mushroom Soup with Crumbled Bacon

Preparation Time **: 15 minutes**

Cooking Time :55 minutes

Servings **: 8**

Ingredients **:**

- 1 Tablespoon of lard
- 1 and ½ lbs. of white mushrooms
- 1/2 cup of water
- 1/2 cups of almond milk
- 2 green onions, finely sliced
- 3 sprigs of fresh rosemary
- 2 cloves garlic, finely chopped
- slices of bacon, fried and crumbled
- **Salt and ground black pepper**

Directions **:**

1. Heat the lard in a large skillet and sauté green onions and garlic over medium-high heat.
2. Season with the salt and pepper, and rosemary; pour water and cook for 5 minutes.
3. Add the mushrooms and sauté for 1-2 minutes.

4. Pour the almond milk, stir, cover and simmer for 40 minutes over low heat.
5. Remove the rosemary and transfer the soup in your blender; blend until creamy and soft.
6. Adjust salt, and if necessary, add some warm water.
7. Chop the bacon and fry in a hot pan until it becomes crisp.
8. **Serve your soup in bowls and sprinkle with chopped bacon.**

Nutrition:

- Calories 130
- Fat 3.9 g
- Carbohydrates 21.2 g
- Sugar 10.4 g
- Protein 3.9 g
- Cholesterol 6 mg

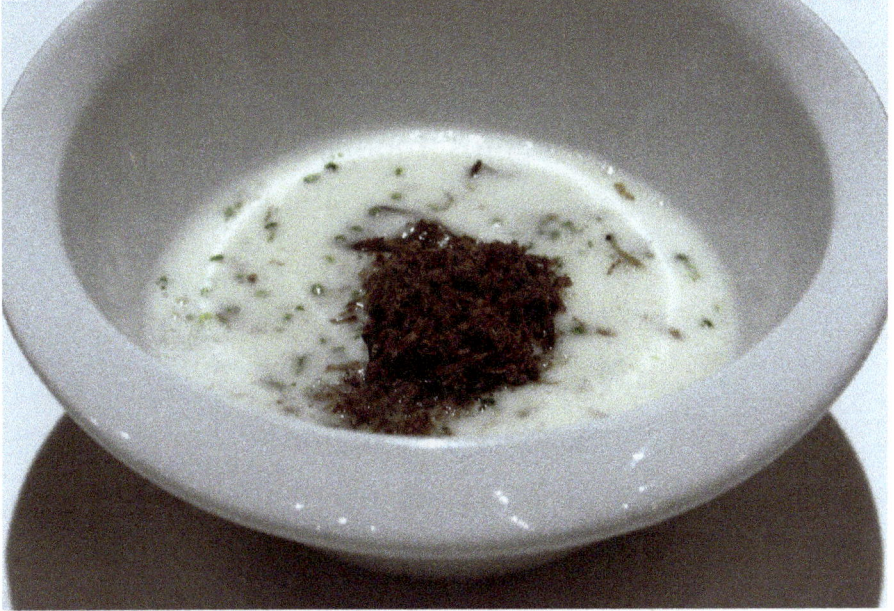

Creamy Mushroom and Zucchini Soup

Preparation and Cooking time: **40 minutes**

Servings **: 8**

Ingredients:

- 1 large zucchini, chopped
- 1 lb. fresh mushrooms, chopped
- 3 cups chicken or vegetable stock
- 1 medium onion, chopped
- 2 cloves garlic, minced
- 2 bay leaves
- 1 tablespoon dried thyme
- 1 tablespoon ghee
- 1 cup coconut milk
- Sea salt
- Freshly ground black pepper

Directions **:**

1. Place a large saucepan over medium heat and melt the ghee. Add the onions and garlic. Sauté about 3 minutes.

2. Add the mushrooms, bay leaves, and thyme. Cook an additional 4 minutes.

3. Add the zucchini and cook until the vegetables release their juices.

4. Add the stock to the pan and bring it to a boil. Reduce the heat and let it simmer about 5 minutes.

5. Discard the bay leaves and add the coconut milk. Simmer another 5 minutes, stirring the mixture frequently.

6. **Transfer the soup to a blender in batches and process until smooth. If you have an immersion blender, you can use it. Serve warm.**

Nutrition:

- Calories 195
- Fat 11.2 g
- Carbohydrates 20.1 g
- Sugar 4.3 g
- Protein 5.5 g
- Cholesterol 0 mg

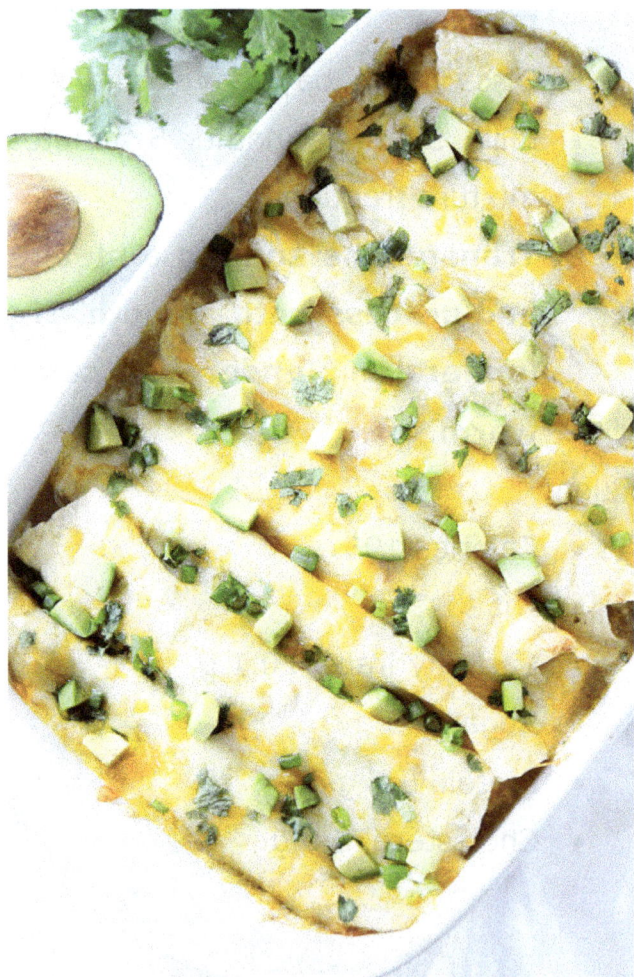

Creamy Cauliflower Chowder

Preparation and Cooking Time **: 20-25 minutes**

Servings **: 8**

Ingredients **:**

- 1 head of cauliflower cut into small florets
- ¾ cup diced carrots
- ½ cup diced onion
- 1 cup milk
- 1 tablespoon butter
- ¼ cup cream cheese
- 5 cloves of garlic, minced
- ½ teaspoon dried oregano
- 1 teaspoon freshly ground pepper
- salt to taste
- 1 cup of water
- 1 tablespoon of olive oil and 3 oz of shredded cheddar cheese for topping

Directions **:**

1. Heat butter in a soup pot.
2. Add onion and garlic and sauté for a few minutes.

3. Add cauliflower, carrots, milk, pepper, salt, and oregano.
4. Bring this mixture to boil and then reduce heat to a simmer.
5. After the cauliflower is tender, remove soup pot from heat and pour the mixture into a blender.
6. Blend soup until creamy then pour it back in the pot.
7. Add a cup of water along with cream cheese.
8. Simmer for 5 to 10 minutes and then turn off heat.
9. **Top with olive oil and shredded cheddar.**

Nutrition:

- Calories 208
- Fat 10.4 g
- Carbohydrates 6.3 g
- Sugar 4.1 g
- Protein 21.7 g
- Cholesterol 33 mg

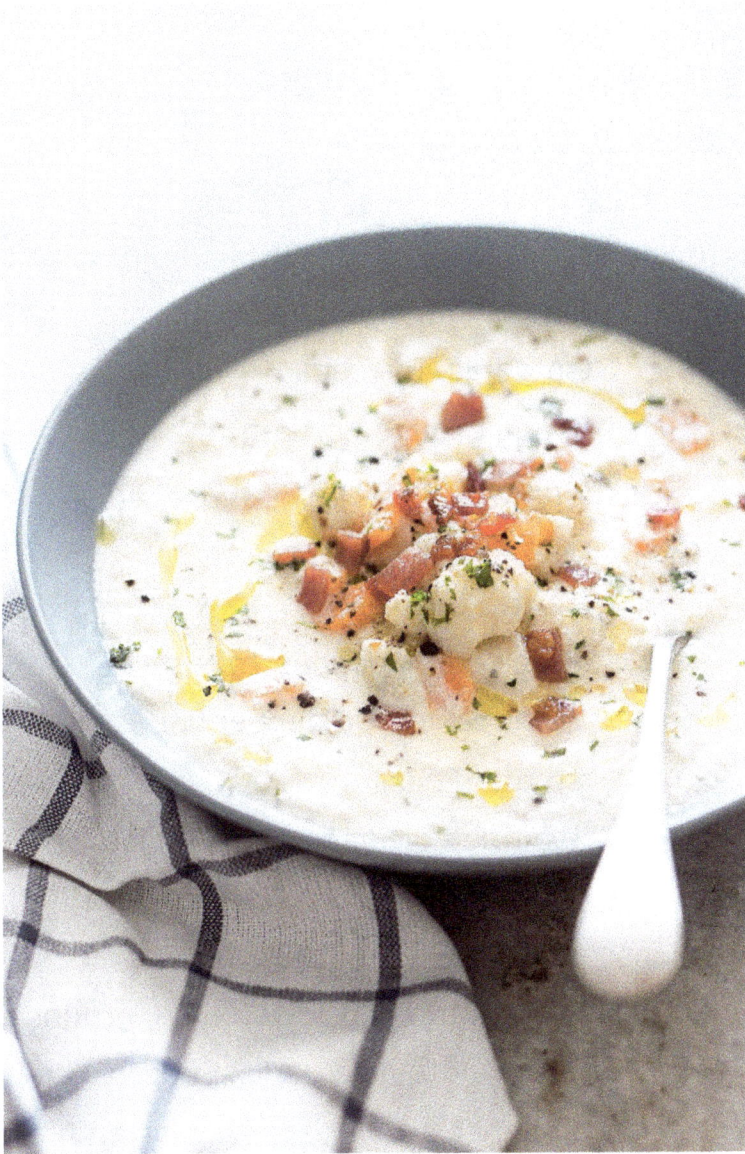

Chicken Meatloaf Cups with Pancetta

Preparation Time: **10 minutes**

Cooking Time :25 minutes

Servings **: 6**

Ingredients

- 2 tbsp onion, chopped
- 1 tsp garlic, minced
- 1 pound ground chicken
- 2 ounces cooked pancetta, chopped
- 1 egg, beaten
- 1 tsp mustard
- Salt and black pepper, to taste
- ½ tsp crushed red pepper flakes
- 1 tsp dried basil
- ½ tsp dried oregano
- **4 ounces cheddar cheese, cubed**

Directions

1. In a bowl, mix mustard, onion, ground chicken, egg, pancetta, and garlic. Season with oregano, red pepper, black pepper, basil and salt.

2. Split the mixture into greased muffin cups. Lower one cube of cheddar cheese into each meatloaf cup.

3. Close the top to cover the cheese. Bake in the oven at 345ºF for 20 minutes, or until the meatloaf cups become golden brown.

4. **Let cool for 10 minutes before transferring from the muffin pan.**

Nutrition:

- Calories 237
- Fat 4.5 g
- Carbohydrates 37.5 g
- Sugar 1.9 g
- Protein 13.2 g
- **Cholesterol 0 mg**

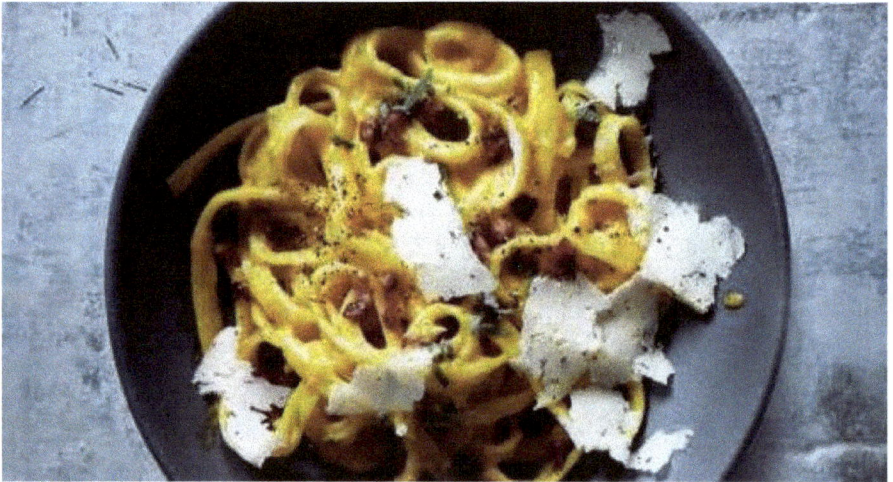

Ham and Emmental Eggs

Preparation Time **: 10 minutes**

Cooking Time :35 minutes

Servings **: 6**

Ingredients

- 1 tbsp olive oil
- 4 slices ham, chopped
- ½ cup chives, chopped
- ½ cup broccoli, chopped
- 1 clove garlic, minced
- 1 tsp fines herbs
- ¼ cup vegetable broth
- 5 eggs
- **1 ½ cups Emmental cheese, shredded**

Directions

1. In a frying pan, warm oil. Add in ham and cook for 4 minutes, until brown and crispy; set aside.

2. Using the same pan, cook chives. Place in the garlic and broccoli and cook until soft as you stir occasionally. Stir in broth and fines herbs and cook for 6 more minutes.

3. Make 5 holes in the mixture until you are able to see the bottom of your pan.

4. Crack an egg into each hole. Spread cheese over the top and cook for 6 more minutes. Scatter the reserved ham over to serve.

Nutrition:

- Calories 450
- Fat 4.3 g
- Carbohydrates 72.6 g
- Sugar 2.6 g
- Protein 29.9 g
- **Cholesterol 19 mg**

www.ingramcontent.com/pod-product-compliance
Lightning Source LLC
Chambersburg PA
CBHW050751030426
42336CB00012B/1763